A Prescription for Your Healthcare Survival
An Insider's Look into Healthcare in the 21st Century

By

Debra C. Camejo R. N.

Legg family Reunion
2009
Best of Health

Debbie

The purpose of this book is to provide the reader with information and tips to be used to seek out the best medical care for themselves and their loved ones. This book is not intended as a substitute for professional or legal advice. Readers are advised to seek the counsel and treatment of a licensed medical physician or legal counsel when appropriate. The author and publisher specifically disclaim any and all responsibility for any adverse effects arising from the use of information contained within these pages or failing to follow medical advice offered from a treating physician.

Published by
Camcorp LLC
camcorp@earthlink.net

Cover design by Debra C. Camejo
Cover graphics by Jeremy Robinson
Interior Design and typesetting by Camcorp LLC
Editor: Diane J. Ploch
Cover Photograph used by permission of Camcorp LLC

Printed and bound in the United States
Lightning Source Inc. trade paperback 2008
Lightning Source Inc. (US)
1246 Heil Quaker Blvd.
La Vergne, TN USA 37086
E-mail: inquiry@lightningsource.com
Voice: (615) 213-5815
Fax: (615) 213-4725

First Edition
Library of Congress
ISBN-13
978-0-615-22356-8

Dedication

To Skip and Chris for all your patience and understanding throughout the past few years. Your love and support are what keeps me going.

To my mentor and special friend, Dr. Gerard J. Foye, who set the bar for the standards for excellence in patient care and brought me back from the brink of death, on more than one occasion.

In our Hearts forever, Mom and Joyce - 2006.

Acknowledgments

There are so many people I'd like to acknowledge. I have been supported and encouraged by my loving husband, son, and close friends during some of the most tumultuous years of my life. I can always count on my husband to be there to hold my hand when I am ill, pick up the pieces of my life or drop whatever he is doing to support me. His continued support means more to me than he will ever know. The love and encouragement of my family and friends make it possible for me to get up each day and put one foot in front of the other and keep moving forward.

I'd like to acknowledge my Aunt Adeline, a lifelong career nurse who dedicated her life to caring for others. She was truly my inspiration for becoming a nurse. I followed her footsteps by attending the same nursing school. Adeline has always been like a second mother to me.

I'd like to thank Cousin El, Laurie, Lin, Terri, Sue Mat, Barb, Mary W., Marie, Val, Karolee, Dorothy, Wilma, Tuna and Sandy for their love and support during the past years. I couldn't have made it without you in my life. To my Maine friends, Dr. Will and Mary for sharing some of the issues encountered by physicians in the workplace.

My mother taught me the basics of love, honesty, integrity and forgiveness. She was a woman of incredible strength, will and spirit, who believed in family and all that is good in people. She always put her family and friends needs before her own.

As her health deteriorated, she insisted that she was fine and "not that bad." It took all her courage and fortitude to learn how to walk again after a devastating injury due to a medication reaction. I stood by her side and proudly watched her struggle to take those first steps. Time and time again, she overcame drastic changes in her

i

body and defied her doctors' dire predictions. As each medical visit brought severe challenges, she surmounted what seemed impossible odds. I was astounded by her strength, determination, and aplomb. She fought so many illnesses and injuries and never complained. She quietly just kept pushing forward with a smile on her face.

I miss gossiping with her, her hugs and advice. It turns out, she was the glue that truly held our family together. She went on ahead where there are no doctors, no medication and no pain. I love and miss her. I strive to be my mother's daughter every day, one in which she would be proud.

Also, in memory of my sister-in-law, Joyce, a loving wife, daughter, sister and mother, who fiercely loved and protected her two children. She fought and lost a difficult and painful battle with cancer. She tried to protect those around her from the devastating pain and changes that ravaged her body and spirit. I miss our hour-long phone calls to chat about all of life's problems and how we resolved to conquer them together.

I'd like to thank Lea, for her support and for her insight as a new graduate nurse in 2007.

On the technical side, I have to thank Korin Kendra, Ph.D., for her inspiration and advice in my first venture in book writing and publishing. Kori was brave enough to go down the road ahead of me with her first published novel, "Coffee House Affairs."

I'd also like to thank my editor/proofreader Diane J. Ploch, for her patience, guidance, commitment and friendship throughout the rewriting process. I feel blessed to have gotten to know you better this past year. I wish I had paid more attention in English class! And yes, I can type as fast as I can talk.

Jeremy Robinson, a published author in his own right, has also been invaluable with his guidance and suggestions as well as being my graphic design artist.

Gary C. Elliott, CPA, has been invaluable with the monetary side of this venture. Gary knew exactly what needed to be done, how and why. He was ever so patient with my repeated phone calls.

Thank you to all who shared their stories with me and allowed me to share them with others so that we can all be better health consumers.

And of course I have to thank my team of doctors who keep me going. I have chosen you and keep going to you because of the trust and relationship that I have developed with you. Thank you for caring for me even when I haven't been the best patient!

Parts adapted from Eulogy of Helen M. Cooper - written by Lauren Cooper Clemons.

Introduction

I graduated from nursing school in the 1970s. My parents had encouraged me to continue my schooling and become a physician. However, as much as I loved the field of medicine, I wanted to marry, have children and was eager to use my new knowledge as a registered nurse. I had worked for several years as a nurse's aide prior to nursing school and felt that I had a good idea of what nursing involved. After graduation, and awaiting my state nursing board results, I worked as a private nurse in a home, caring for one patient. Soon my state board results arrived and I embarked on my career and journey as a registered nurse in a hospital setting. I worked at the same hospital for 17 years.

It has now been several years since I left hospital employment. I had been injured on the job with a fractured vertebra. My employer failed to diagnose and treat my injury over a period of a year and a half. Subsequently, I was forced to leave my position due to health reasons. I helped orchestrate the care for my father at home for 10 years as Parkinson's disease slowly robbed him of the everyday functions of his body, system by system. My mother followed, as she battled severe congestive obstructive pulmonary disease (COPD), heart and circulatory issues that lead to her death in the fall of 2006. I helped to coordinate her care through many long hospitalizations over the past several years. During her hospitalizations, I observed the medical professionals at work and became increasingly frustrated at the lack of care, time and physical assessment provided to my mother. When my mother was transferred to a rehabilitation facility, the hands-on care with licensed professionals was even less.

One year after my mother's death, I was sitting in a doctor's waiting room. I noticed two women sitting close by in chairs, one of whom I recognized. I had worked with the younger woman, a registered nurse, about 23 years ago. I approached her and we began a conversation. She was there with her elderly aunt who had some evidence of Alzheimer's. She stated that she had also recently assisted her mother-in-law when she was hospitalized for a broken hip at the same hospital where we had both worked. I made a comment about her family being fortunate to have her assist them with their medical needs as I had for mine. I shouldn't have been surprised to hear her tell me about what she perceived to be the lack of care in the hospital and how she was accused by a nurse manager of "looking for trouble" while trying to get the best care for her family member. That was when I knew that all the emotions and feelings that I had felt over the past several years were valid. I had come face to face with hospital administration trying to get them to provide my mother with basic nursing care, trying to alert the staff of risk factors to prevent complications and inform them of my mother's individual needs. It all seemed to fall on deaf ears.

By reading this book, I hope readers will learn how to interact with physicians and nurses to get the best care for themselves and their loved ones.

Table of Contents

Prologue

First Do No Harm. These are the words most people associate with the Hippocratic Oath taken by physicians.

The oath, attributed to Hippocrates, the father of medicine, goes as such:

"I swear by Apollo Physician and Asclepius and Hygeia and Panaceia and all the gods and goddesses, making them my witnesses, that I will fulfill according to my ability and judgment this oath and this covenant: To hold him who has taught me this art as equal to my parents and to live my life in partnership with him, and if he is in need of money to give him a share of mine, and to regard his offspring as equal to my brothers in male lineage and to teach them this art - if they desire to learn it - without fee and covenant; to give a share of precepts and oral instruction and all the other learning to my sons and to the sons of him who has instructed me and to pupils who have signed the covenant and have taken an oath according to the medical law, but no one else.

I will apply dietetic measures for the benefit of the sick according to my ability and judgment; I will keep them from harm and injustice.

I will neither give a deadly drug to anybody who asked for it, nor will I make a suggestion to this effect. Similarly I will not give to a woman an abortive remedy. In purity and holiness I will guard my life and my art.

I will not use the knife, not even on sufferers from stone, but will withdraw in favor of such men as are engaged in this work.

Whatever houses I may visit, I will come for the benefit of the sick, remaining free of all intentional injustice, of all mischief and in particular of sexual relations with both female and male persons, be they free or slaves.

What I may see or hear in the course of the treatment or even outside of the treatment in regard to the life of men, which on no account one must spread abroad, I will keep to myself, holding such things shameful to be spoken about.

If I fulfill this oath and do not violate it, may it be granted to me to enjoy life and art, being honored with fame among all men for all time to come; if I transgress it and swear falsely, may the opposite of all this be my lot." (1)

Likewise, nurses take the Nightingale Pledge. Florence Nightingale was a woman born in the 19th century who devoted herself to the caring of others when nursing was equated with that of cook or maid. The Nightingale Pledge goes as such:

"The Nightingale Pledge was composed by a committee chaired by Lystra Gretter, an instructor of nursing at the old Harper Hospital in Detroit, Michigan, and was first used by its graduating class in the spring of 1893:

- I solemnly pledge myself before God and in the presence of this assembly, to pass my life in purity and to practice my profession faithfully.

- I will abstain from whatever is deleterious and mischievous, and will not take or knowingly administer any harmful drug.

- I will do all in my power to maintain and elevate the standard of my profession, and will hold in confidence all personal matters committed to my keeping and all family affairs coming to my knowledge in the practice of my calling.

- With loyalty will I endeavor to aid the physician, in his work, and devote myself to the welfare of those committed to my care." (2)

Chapter 1

WHO's WHO

"As it takes two to make a quarrel, so it takes two to make a disease, the microbe and its host." - Charles V. Chapin

Physicians are truly devoted people who spend many years of their adulthood in schooling and training to be able to practice medicine.

TRAINING, QUALIFICATIONS AND ADVANCEMENT

The formal education and training for physicians are amongst the most demanding of any occupation. Four years of undergraduate school (college), followed by four years of medical school, the first two of which are typically spent in a classroom and two additional years working under a physician in a hospital or other health care setting. After four years in medical school, the person will attain a degree in either Medicine (M.D.) or Osteopathy (D.O.).

The first year of practice after graduation from medical school is the internship year. Many go on to complete an additional three to eight years of internship and residency, depending on the specialty selected. Most medical schools offer a customary eight years of training, although a few offer a combined undergraduate and medical school program lasting six years.

Undergraduate students may obtain their degree in physics, biology, mathematics, English, or chemistry. Students also take courses in the humanities and the social sciences. The minimum educational requirement for entry into a medical school is three years of college; most applicants, however, have at least a bachelor's degree. Entrance or admission into a top medical school is very competitive. For this reason, a fair number go out of the country for training. However, upon graduation, they still need to meet U.S. standards if they intend to practice medicine in the United States.

There are many types of physicians, with varied training. It is wise to investigate a physician to whom you will be entrusting your health care. The most common types of physicians and surgeons are defined on the following pages.

PHYSICIAN

Physician in the broad sense, usually in North America, applies to any legally qualified and licensed practitioner of medicine. In the United States, the term physician is now commonly used to describe any medical doctor holding the Doctor of Medicine (M.D.) or Doctor of Osteopathic Medicine (D.O.) degree.

Both M.D.s and D.O.s may use accepted methods of treatment, including drugs and surgery, while D.O.s place special emphasis on the body's musculoskeletal system, preventive medicine and holistic patient care. The American Medical Association, established 1847, uses the word physician in this broad sense to describe all its members. (3) In North America, we use the word "physician" as synonymous with "doctor."

However, not all doctors have a degree in medicine. A person who has achieved a degree in philosophy (PhD) may also be referred to as doctor. Doctorate degrees can be attained in many other fields as well, including, but not limited to, engineering, law, geology, theology and even nursing. I remember reading about a possible restriction of the use of the title of "Dr." a few years ago. Some wanted to limit the use for medical doctors only to avoid confusion with those who have a doctorate in another field of study. To my knowledge, no legislation has been passed to that effect. I do believe that similar legislation has been passed in Ontario, Canada, that only allows medical physicians, dentists and optometrists to be referred to as "Doctor."

SURGEON

In medicine, a surgeon is a person who performs surgery. Surgery is a broad category of invasive medical treatment that involves cutting of a body, whether human or other organism. Surgeons may be physicians, dentists or veterinarians who specialize in surgery. (4)

There are many specialties within the field of surgery. Some surgeons prefer to remain general surgeons who can operate on any given part of the anatomy. Others prefer to specialize in certain areas of the anatomy, which I will break down later in this chapter.

OSTEOPATHS, PODIATRISTS, CHIROPRACTORS AND NATUROPATHIC PHYSICIANS

Within the United States, the term physician may also describe Doctor of Osteopathic medicine (D.O.) who are licensed physicians. However, outside the USA, osteopaths are recognized as physicians in only 48 countries. Primary care physicians can hold degrees such as Doctor of Chiropractic (D.C.), Doctor of

Naturopathic Medicine (N.D.) or Doctors of Podiatric Medicine (D.P.M.). These physicians maintain a narrow scope of practice compared to Medical Doctors and Osteopaths. (5)

There are many different fields in medicine. All require their own level of expertise. During training, doctors are exposed to all of these areas, but then must continue their education if they want to specialize. As the field of medicine has become increasingly specialized, so have the titles. I have included some of the more popular ones here:

Anesthetics

General practice

Medicine

Obstetrics and Gynecology

Ophthalmology

Pediatrics

Pathology

Plastic Surgery

Psychiatry

Radiology

Surgery (Including Dental Surgery)

There are many medical specialists and some of the fields of medicine in which they work are included below. Doctors can work in one or more specialties.

Cardiologists (heart)

Dermatologist (skin)

Endocrinologist (glands)

Gastroenterologist (digestive)

Gynecologist (female reproductive system)

Hematologist (blood)

Maxillofacial (jaws, mouth, face)

Neonatologist (newborns)

Nephrologist (kidney)

Neurologist (nervous system)

Obstetrician (Childbirth)

Oncologist (cancer)

Otologist (ear)

Ophthalmologist (eyes)

Orthopedic (bones, joints)

Otolaryngologist (ear, nose, throat)

Pediatrician (children)

Perinatologist (High risk mother/fetus)

Proctologist (colon)

Podiatrist (feet)

Pulmonologist (lungs)

Psychiatrist (mental)

Rheumatologist (arthritis)

Thoracic Specialist (chest)

Urologist (bladder/urinary tract)

Residents, either medical or surgical, are doctors in training. A medical resident has a medical degree and is in a stage of post-graduate training, in the chosen medical specialty. They must work under a licensed physician during this period. Some residents have completed the internship year, while others include the first year of residency as the internship year. Most are required to complete four years of a residency.

State regulations can vary regarding continuing education for licensed M.D.s. Some require yearly continuing medical education credits while others have a more relaxed schedule. In addition to state regulations, each hospital or professional organization may have their own requirements regarding continuing medical education credits.

Chapter 2

CHECKING CREDENTIALS

"No man is a good doctor who has never been sick himself." - Chinese Proverb

Now that you know the different types of physicians, you need to be able to check out your doctor's credentials and understand a little more about his or her training. Proper training and credentials can be critical when choosing a physician or surgeon. This issue made the news when Donya West, the mother of Kanye West, a well-known hip hop musician, died after complications of cosmetic surgery in late 2007. The procedure was performed by a surgeon who was not certified by the American Board of Plastic Surgery. He had been sued twice for medical malpractice in the year 2000 and ordered to pay almost $500,000. (6) The surgeon you choose should be board certified in the field of surgery that you or a loved one is about to undergo. This in itself is never a guarantee, however, that medical or surgical complications will be avoided. Things can and do go wrong. Many times it has no bearing on the physician or his training. There are many factors that can have an adverse effect on surgery. The patient's own health and vices can seriously affect the outcome of surgery or the healing process. Fortunately, most people are helped by their physicians and most physicians have good intentions and skills.

The medical license, medical school and year of graduation of any surgeon, physician, nurse or other licensed professional can be checked with the state medical board or licensing board in the state in which they are licensed to practice.

There are several sources for checking a physician's credentials, in addition to the state licensing board. Other methods may include checking for board certification, word of mouth from friends and family or some that I have listed below. Connecticut Magazine, New York Magazine, and U.S. News and World Report have all done feature articles regarding choices of "Top Docs." Castle Connolly Medical, LTD, has published a book entitled, "Top Doctors in the New York Metropolitan Area," which is available in the reference section of several libraries that I checked in the tri-state area. I am not sure if other areas of the country are following suit with regional reference books, but it would be worthwhile to check. Castle Connolly's Web site at: www.castleconnolly.com also offers a Doctor Disciplinary Link Search for the 50 States. The Doctor Disciplinary link allows you to search your State licensing board for a physician by name. It will list any reported malpractice settlements in addition to complaints or actions on the part of the State Medical Board against the physician.

You can access the New York Magazine list of over 1,400 Top Doctors in the New York City region at their Web site: http://nymag.com/bestdoctors/.

Likewise, Connecticut Magazine has several editions of Top Docs in various specialties on their Web site. See the Resources Information section at the end of this book for Web site address and further information.

The physicians' in these magazines were chosen by their colleagues for inclusion into the Top Docs category. Again, this system for choosing the "Top Docs" is not perfect. I have worked alongside some of these Connecticut Top Docs and have networked with other nurses, who would disagree with some of those who made the list. The reverse is also true. There are many intelligent, devoted, compassionate doctors that have never made the list. So again, you may want to check their educational background, their board certification and set up an appointment to meet with the physician personally. You will have to decide for yourself if your personality works well with the chosen physician.

RateMD's (www.Ratemds.com) is another Web site that allows patients to rate their doctors. Again, this would have to be used with some caution. You may find only those extremely satisfied or unsatisfied taking the time to rate their doctors on this Web site and you may not get an accurate picture. This is only a small fraction of some of the reasons why you should choose one physician over another.

Vitals.com is a Web site that was launched in January 2008. This site provides consumers with physician background information such as schooling, board certification, publications and malpractice suits. Presently, there are over 720,000 physicians listed on the Web site. Consumers can also rate a physician on this site.

Zagat Survey, known for rating hotels, eateries and entertainment linked up with Wellpoint and Blue Cross in January 2008. They have instituted a 30 point assessment scale used by members on their respective Web sites to rate physicians. Members of Wellpoint and Anthem in Los Angeles, Connecticut and Southern Ohio currently are able to share their physician experience, either positive or negative, with other members. Members need to create an account at www.anthem.com. Click on the tab for the provider finder. A search can be initiated either by provider, location or physician name. After a physician's name is located, click on "more information." To add your own review, click on "add your review" and rate your physician. This service is not available to the general public who are not covered by these health care insurance plans.

Chapter 3

MEDICAL TERMINOLOGY

"Primum est non nocere - First, Do No Harm." - Hippocrates

The field of medicine has its own language. Much of it is based on Latin. Most physicians want their patients to understand their treatment. Patients who understand their treatment appear to be more compliant and may have better long-term results. Never hesitate to have a doctor repeat information to you that you do not understand, whether it is regarding to treatment, diagnosis or any other aspect of your medical care. A friend in my neighborhood occasionally stops by to update me on her relative's medical condition. His physician had informed the patient that he had "a five centimeter polyp in his bladder." The daughter looked at the doctor and said, "Speak English." She simply did not understand if five centimeters was the size of a pea or the size of a grapefruit. And was a polyp cancerous, she wondered? There are some physicians and surgeons who simply don't or won't "speak English." If you repeatedly ask for interpretation and cannot get any satisfactory answers, it may be time to find a new doctor.

If you have made repeated attempts, but are unable to communicate with your physician or surgeon and feel that this interferes with your care, hopefully, you are in a situation to change. If not, bring someone with you to the appointment that is familiar with medical terminology. I have experienced this with one of my mother's surgeons, who "on paper" had a stellar training in his medical specialty. He, however, did not feel the need to communicate his findings, treatment or any other aspect of care to my mother or myself. Fortunately, my mother was able to pick and choose her physicians and surgeons and did not have an insurance plan with a gatekeeper or point of service plan where the patient can only go to participating physicians. I understand that not everyone is so fortunate. Perhaps a trusted family physician would be willing to step in as an intermediary and translate any lacking information. If the surgeon employs a licensed nurse or physician assistant in his office, it may be beneficial to have them review your illness and treatment plan with you in terms that you can understand.

Prescriptions written by your physician are based on Latin abbreviations. Unless you have a medical background, it can be difficult to read. Fortunately, pharmacists are responsible for transcribing the information onto your prescription label in language that you can understand. I have included some common prescription abbreviations below. You may want to take a minute to read your prescription prior to handing it over to your pharmacist to compare the information that is written on the label. Even pharmacists occasionally have difficulty reading a physician's handwriting!

disp. = dispense

sig. = let it be labeled

a.c. = before meals

p.c. = after meals

q.d. = every day

q.o.d. = every other day

b.i.d. = twice a day

t.i.d.= three times a day

q.i.d = four times a day

q. h.s. = every night

q.2. h. = every 2 hours

p.o. = by mouth

gtt. = drop

o.d.= right eye

o.s. = left eye

mg. = milligram

mcg. = microgram

d.a.w. = dispense as written

caps. = capsules

tabs.= tablets

p.r.n. = as needed

i = one

ii = two

iii = three

Chapter 4

YOUR PHYSICIAN'S TIME

"Healing is a matter of time, but it is sometimes also a matter of opportunity." - Hippocrates

Physicians are busy people. Many of today's healthcare institutions are employing physicians as "groups" to see patients. This can benefit the physician who otherwise may not be able to afford the high cost of malpractice insurance which can run anywhere from the high thousands to hundreds of thousands per year. However, group physicians working for a healthcare institution may have to abide by patient ratios set by the institution. This means that the institution can mandate the number of patients that a physician sees in any given day. This situation occurred to a physician of mine who had treated me for 16 years at a prestigious teaching hospital. She was told she had to see more patients per day. As a specialist, healer, teacher of new physicians, world lecturer and medical researcher, her time was already compromised. She chose to

29

leave the institution and enter into a different practice, where I still see her today.

Added to the time constraints of physicians is the necessity to keep up with continued learning in their field and the need to adapt to constant changes in the field of medicine. The technology is ever changing and much of a physician's time is spent keeping abreast of the changes. Physicians in private practice must also factor in the management and costs of running a private practice. Rising costs of malpractice insurance, salary and benefits for ancillary staff as well as building costs and maintenance must be factored in. The physician must work longer and harder to keep his business afloat.

Even the routine of record keeping can take a lot of a physician's limited time. A physician that I visited was unhappy with a new system instituted in his office to chart electronically. Fortunately, the physician was computer literate, but now he had to take his laptop into each examination room to the patient. His complaint was "now I spend my time talking to a computer and not to the patient." As he interviewed me, he sat and typed my responses into the computer. Much of the same information had to be entered more than once, sometimes up to three times. Many of these medical documentation programs are generic. They are not individualized to the patient or the medical specialty that they are used to gather information on. Patients with complex medical problems may not be conducive to this type of charting. I shiver to think about the information on the laptop being lost or stolen. Stolen computer databases are already an occurrence in the United Kingdom. Databases containing personal information have also been stolen here in the United States from my own state's Department of Motor Vehicles. Laptop computers with personal information have been stolen from office buildings and locked cars. Hopefully, your physician's electronic files are encrypted and password protected. Secure computers and networks are vital to keeping our personal information safe. Hiring a professional company to monitor a hospital's electronic charting and electronic records can be expensive, but well worth the expense when so much personal information is at risk. Many smaller physician practices may forgo the security updates and scans that ensure patient privacy to save money. However, if electronic records and charting are here to stay, security must be given the highest priority.

With the advent of electronic charting, steps are being taken within the hospital to discourage hospital employees from electronically looking at information that is not relevant to their own patients. Some hospitals have already fired employees for doing so and are utilizing tracking software to watch employee computer usage.

In February 2008, Google Inc., a search engine on the Internet, announced that it would begin storing individual medical records on a Web site. The information would be password protected and not open to the public. A health profile would be created for those who participated to include medical history, allergies and medications taken. Currently, the pilot project is using patients from the Cleveland Clinic who volunteer to use the service. The Cleveland Clinic already uses a similar system called "My Chart." (7)

A different physician I visited was also using a new electronic charting system. He stated that it was a standardized computer program, not as efficient and not as individualized as paper charts. He did say that it was easier for others to read (no kidding, with doctors' handwriting as it is!)

At another medical facility a physician I visited also had made the change to electronic records. I was dismayed to see all of my personal information on the screen, including my Social Security number. I did make a request to have my Social Security number removed from the screen. There is no need for anyone but the billing department to have that for insurance purposes, although Social Security numbers are no longer used for most health care insurance identification numbers. I had to speak with several people, but eventually, my Social Security number was removed from the screen.

A newly graduated registered nurse working in a large, local metropolitan hospital has been using electronic charting on the busy medical unit where she is assigned. She states that electronic charting does not save time, a lot of double charting occurs and the charts are not linked to the emergency room charting. So when a patient is admitted through the emergency room, a new chart has to be initiated. This can lead to omission of important information and inefficient use of time.

During a personal visit to a local emergency room in June 2008, I noted the physician sitting in front of a computer screen for approximately thirty minutes and at the bedside for five minutes. The wait to get into the emergency treatment area was approximately two hours. Documentation is important, but the current electronic charting does appear to be slowing some physicians down.

The use of electronic records and charting has been slow to gain popularity. Most physicians cite affordability, value, finding the appropriate program and fear of quick obsolescence according to a survey in the June 2003 issue of the New England Journal of Medicine. The survey highlighted some of the positive aspects of electronic records and charting. Some of these include a reduction in errors, improvement in communication and access to monitoring medication safety.

YOUR PHYSICIAN VISITS

Physicians are busy people. Many physicians today report rushed patient care, lower level of pay, increased paperwork, increased overhead expenses and less control over treatment. The field of medicine has vastly changed in the past 100 years with increased technology, increased involvement of medical insurance companies and less single physician medical practices.

Each physician typically allots 15 minutes of his scheduled time for a patient. So what does this mean to the patient? It means we have to be more prepared when we go to the doctor. He may not be able to see or access all of our past medical history at his fingertips if he is looking at a computer screen. You can help him by bringing copies of your past medical reports, a list of your medications, a list of your issues to be discussed and be prepared to tell him any relevant issues that are concerning you that he may have forgotten. He is seeing many people over the course of the day and cannot remember everything about everyone.

It may be helpful to bring the following with you to your appointment or your yearly physical:

- A list of questions and concerns. Always discuss the most urgent question first. Most people will put off the most embarrassing or pressing question until the end.

- A list of your current medications with dosing information.
- Your health history, including a copy for your doctor.
- Any pertinent information, such as - home blood pressure readings, blood glucose readings, etc.
- A copy of your family health history.

One physician that I visited years ago scheduled three patients for the same appointment time. I knew this by asking the other two patients in the waiting room. Sure enough, we were all escorted into three adjoining rooms at the same time. Dr. G. entered room # 1, asked what the complaints were, told the patient to undress and exited the room. He proceeded to room # 2, and did the same and then into room # 3 for another round. Then he returned to room #1 for the physical examination, and seemed a little confused about why I was there. And it went on and on in this manner until he finished with all three. I felt that I was only getting partial attention and did not feel that this environment suited my needs. I returned once more, only to be subjected to the same door game. So it was time for me to show myself the door and move on to another physician.

Creating a copy of your health history has never been easier. Home computers make it easy to create a health history and update it periodically. Many online resources are also creating blank health history sheets that simply need to be downloaded and answered.

Zebrahealth.com has a Personal Health Record that can be completed and downloaded from the Internet to bring to your physician appointment.

Doctor office visits can be challenging - beginning with the call to make the appointment! Not all office staff is created equally and I am sad to say that I have had my fair share of encounters with rude office staff that have little or no medical training. I have had many others tell me of similar situations. These women (yes, I know there are some men) who answer the phone are in control and you are at their mercy. The staff who answer the telephone act as gatekeepers determining who gets in and who gets to talk to whom. This can be very frustrating if you have a serious problem that needs urgent care. If you experience problems with the person who answers your physician's telephone, and you have an urgent situation, ask for the office nurse or the physician to call you back immediately. Ask when you can expect a return phone call. After your situation is resolved, be sure to inform the physician if you consistently experience difficulty with his office staff. The office nurse should have more medical knowledge and help you obtain an appointment, a phone call back from the doctor or direct you to the assistance that you need. If you are unable to get satisfaction with a phone call, never hesitate to go to an Emergency Room if you perceive this to be a serious health problem that may be life threatening.

Fortunately, there are a lot of wonderful men and women without medical training that answer these phones, too. Most will screen your calls as if their life depended on it. Phone calls from one doctor to another go a long way in getting your foot in the door. Having another close family member (i.e., spouse) already as a patient of that office can also help.

Most ancillary staff in a physician's office are unlicensed. This means they are not registered nurses or licensed practical nurses. They may be medical technicians, patient care technicians, medical assistants, etc. Since 1987, states were required to initiate and maintain nurse's aide training programs and competency evaluations. Prior to that, many were trained "on the job." Your State maintains a registry of certified nurse's aides. As with the telephone receptionists, there are some outstanding, caring and competent people in these positions. Unlicensed staff may perform some office procedures and treatments. Some may have been doing these procedures for years and are very proficient, but I have witnessed errors and have been told of many more.

If you are ever concerned about a blood pressure or other test performed by ancillary staff, please ask your physician to repeat it.

Licensed medical staff can make mistakes, too. I witnessed a pulmonary physician apply a blood pressure cuff upside down and backwards and take a blood pressure reading on my mother. The physician obtained a reading that was well within the parameters of normal. My mother and I had just left an internist's office across the hall where my mother's blood pressure was extremely high and she was being treated for hypertension. My mother and I just looked at each other with a knowing look when the pulmonary doctor told us her reading. (We had to ask, it was not volunteered.)

Of sad note, I had worked with a licensed nurse years ago in the hospital, who had fabricated temperatures, pulses and blood pressures, but recorded them as being done. When co-workers brought the obvious to the attention of hospital administration, the nurse was not reprimanded. I still wonder to this day, why become a nurse if you can't or won't do something as basic as vital signs and what else wasn't this nurse doing? Hopefully, these inept doctors and nurses are few and far between.

A friend of mine was a nursing instructor and then a nurse's aide instructor prior to her retirement several years ago. She worked in a major city in Connecticut. Over time, more and more students were in her class who had their tuition paid for by the State. Her curriculum changed minimally over the years, as she taught the basics or fundamentals of nursing aide care. However, she noted that fewer and fewer students were passing her exams. She also noted students talking on cell phones or appearing to sleep during class with their heads down on their desks. Her life was even threatened at one point and there were students who had a past criminal history. When she reported these issues to upper administration, she was told to "dumb down" the exams so that these students could pass. I shudder to think who will be taking care of me when I need it and it terrifies me to think who is taking care of our elderly and disabled now.

When my mother was hospitalized, I encountered a few "bold" nurse's aides. I made no mention of my nursing degree. Some of these nurse's aides were giving medical advice freely and expected the patients to do as they were told and not question them. Time and time again, I have heard very concerning stories from close friends and relatives who were in a short or long-term nursing facility as a patient. They all told me examples of nurse's aides who would "punish" the patients if they used their call lights too frequently or their personalities were not compatible. Some staff would withhold patient meals until the food was cold, and others' requests for help were simply ignored. Some staff even took it to the extreme by hitting patients. This behavior should never be tolerated. Be sure to keep anecdotal records of names and occurrences, and possibly photographs of any suspected neglect and abuse. Bring it to the attention of the head nurse and the director of nursing. If the situation continues, be prepared to bring it to a state level. If necessary, move the family member out of the facility. If abuse occurs in a Joint Commission on Accreditation of Healthcare Organizations (JACHO) accredited facility a complaint should be filed directly to the Joint Commission. The Joint Commission has an anonymous telephone line and also accepts e-mail complaints. Further information is in the Resources Information section at the end of this book.

Because your physician's office is a busy place, don't assume that no news is good news. If you have not heard back about test results in one or two weeks, be sure to call the office and request them. Medical reports can get lost or misfiled. I have had it personally happen to me. After you obtain your results, ask that a written copy be faxed or mailed to you. This may require you to sign a medical release form. If you know that you are going to request a copy of a test result, some physician's offices will allow you to sign a release prior to the test.

Being prepared for you physician visits should also include being prepared for your future health and welfare. Although no one likes to think of the inevitable, life has been described as being terminal. As we age, it makes good sense to plan for the aging process and possible ill health. Anyone that is a home owner, parent, spouse, or cares about how they would like to be cared for in the event of a sudden, catastrophic illness should prepare well in advance. A Living Will and a Healthcare Power of Attorney are two invaluable legal documents to have. A Living Will lets you choose if you want to be kept alive with advanced medical technology and equipment in the event that you are unable to communicate your wishes. A Healthcare Power of Attorney, or Durable POA for Healthcare will allow you to chose a relative or close friend to direct your health care if you are unable. These documents should be drawn up, signed, witnessed and notarized well in advance of their need. You should make sure that a copy is accessible to your health advocate if you are unable to bring them to the hospital with you. An attorney is the best person to prepare these documents for you. Each state has laws that can differ so be sure to have them prepared in the state in which you reside.

Generational differences between your physician, hospital staff and yourself can also affect your healthcare. In the 21st century, we have 4 generations simultaneously in the workforce. All were raised in different eras with differing values and views of the world.

The youngest generation currently in the work force is in their late teens and early 20's. They are referred to as Generation X. They were born between the years of 1965-1980. This generation like to balance work and play. They are more likely to be open with their sexuality and lifestyles.

Generation Y's were born between 1980 through the year 2000. I see a lot of similarity of these two generations. They grew up being told that they could do anything they wanted, praised for the smallest of accomplishments and expect a free gift in the box when they go to lunch at their favorite fast food restaurant. This generation feels entitled to success and having things their way.

Both these generations are very technologically oriented. They grew up in the computer era and had exposure to cell phones, VCRs, PDAs and video games at a young age. They may be more informal in their attire, attitude and verbal interactions.

The baby boomers were born between 1946-1964. These individuals had to learn vast amounts of new technology as it came along. This group tends to be more individualistic in their thinking. As a patient, they want to know more about their illness and have a say in their choice of treatment. They want to research their illness or diseases to better understand it.

The last group is the mature group over the age of 63 years. This group as a whole tends not to be freethinkers and less technologically advanced. As a patient or nurse, they are less likely to challenge a physician on a diagnosis or treatment.

I have encountered many Generation X and Y employees in the workforce. Time and again, I have noticed the lack of courtesy and respect during these interactions. Upon entering a physician's office, you must sign in or give your name to the receptionist. Many times, members of Generation X or Y will completely ignore you, as you stand right in front of them.

A nursing instructor relayed a story to me of a Generation X woman who was just beginning a registered nursing program at a university. The young woman was required to get signed paperwork back to the instructor by a specific date. The date was approaching fast and the instructor had to remind the young woman. It became apparent that the young woman did not see the need or urgency to inconvenience herself to get the signed papers returned to the instructor. She even suggested that the instructor should go out of her way to come pick up the papers.

I have also heard of a Generation X nurse working in hospital with a large lollypop in her mouth as she went room to room checking her patients. Not so long ago, this would have been considered unprofessional and would never have occurred in a hospital.

Chapter 5

THE PROS AND CONS OF SOCIALIZED MEDICINE

"Realize that the doctor's fight against socialized medicine is your fight. We can't socialize the doctors without socializing the patients" - Ronald Reagan

Socialized medicine is a health care insurance plan for all citizens of a country. The health care coverage is based on a publicly funded system administrated by the government. Some may refer to it as a Universal Health Care system or a National Health Care system. Virtually all of Europe, including the United Kingdom, Canada and Australia, has a National Health Care system.

Many politicians have been promoting socialized medicine as a cure all for the American health care system without identifying all the possible drawbacks.

We currently have programs that are run by the government such as Social Security and Medicare. Both of these programs have serious financial problems and are threatening insolvency in the not so distant future. History has demonstrated that there are hospitals, pharmacies and doctors that are willing to manipulate the system's weaknesses for their own financial gain. Others argue that if the access to medical care is free, more will use it and resources will be stretched beyond their means.

European countries are now in a situation where they have to limit government assistance and access to care. The number of doctors and hospital beds is limited and if more people continue to overuse the system, the costs incurred are higher than the amount the government has allotted.

I have been able to get first hand information from people living in Australia and the United Kingdom regarding their experiences with socialized medicine. A woman in Australia reported to her American friend that she had gallstones and it took two years before they could schedule the removal of her diseased gallbladder.

Residents of the United Kingdom also report long waiting periods for health appointments and pay a National Health Stamp depending on how much they earn. It is deducted from their wages - if they earn enough. A wife can get free treatment on her husband's contributions or a child on his or her parents' contributions. If a person is on "benefit," then it is free. A physician visit under the National Health Service is without any cost to the patient. However, the patient must pay for their own prescriptions.

A distant cousin who lives in England has been writing to me for the past few years about her son's unfortunate accident. Her son John, worked for the Postal Service in the United Kingdom. In November 2004, he was going into the attic when a board fell and hit him very hard on the head. On the day of his accident, John went to the hospital. John suffered bleeding in his brain as a result of the accident and had permanent memory loss as well as other severe physical and mental changes. After the first hospital visit the family paid privately for an appointment with a doctor for follow-up. After that, the family went back to the National Health Service where it took 9 to 12 months just to get an appointment. Sadly, John has permanent disabilities as a result of this accident and has never been able to return to work. He has memory and functional problems, not to mention frustration regarding his medical care. His wife is working so they cannot receive all the help that is necessary, but he does have an Occupational Health Visitor who assesses his physical surroundings for safety. Because of this, he did qualify for some bath aids and grab rails that were installed in his home. In some circumstances, grants are given to add larger bathrooms or more accessible bathrooms in a home; however, the criteria has been changing and making it more difficult for some to qualify.

My cousin in the United Kingdom is also permanently disabled and confined to a wheelchair. Her first wheelchair arrived in 1992 - after waiting for 6 months through the National Health

Service. Can you imagine "waiting" for a wheelchair if you are unable to walk? The National Health Service provided a replacement wheelchair in 2002. In October 2004, she was given an electric wheelchair after waiting five months for it to arrive.

My cousin also has asthma and reports that if she went to the National Health Service she would have to wait between four and six months to get an appointment. Her husband is employed and has his own health coverage. He is able to get an appointment in seven to ten days. They currently pay about 100 British Pounds Sterling or $198.00 (U.S. dollars) to see a private physician. If you are on the National Health Service, the wait for an appointment with a specialist can be months unless a referring physician deems that it is urgent. However, the visit will be free of cost.

Dental care in the United Kingdom is also a challenge. A lot of dentists are no longer participating in the National Health Service. People have to pay privately or travel distances or even go abroad for treatment as it sometimes works out cheaper. If a dentist is participating in the National Health Service, the cost is much cheaper than going to a private dentist. It costs an average of 15.76 in British Pounds Sterling for a dental checkup with a National Health Care participating dentist, which is the approximate of $31.00 (U.S. Dollars). The cost for an amalgam filling would cost about 44 British Pounds Sterling, which is approximately $87.00 (U.S. Dollars).

The fee to see an optician is currently 10 British Pounds Sterling, which is approximately $20.00. According to my British cousin, these fees are all expected to rise soon.

The British National Department of Health was in the news in December 2007, when they "lost" private information of hundreds of thousands of patients who use the free health care system in the United Kingdom. This is reportedly the third such instance where private information has been lost there.

I have heard of stories of excellent care in Europe. My own son lived in the United Kingdom for a year and developed a serious infection. He was fortunate to get immediate care and had to return for several visits. The surgeon, however, was going to cut open the infected site to let it drain when the nurse stepped up to ask the physician if he might like to use a little Novocain before cutting. I have to wonder if this is how they save on costs? Yipes! But the cost for his medical care was free. Another relative was traveling in Europe when she fell on a sidewalk and needed immediate care. She was also treated for free and received excellent emergency care.

I interviewed a young man who was citizen of Canada. He related a health care system similar to that in the United Kingdom. Employees pay a certain percentage of their wages to the government. They can seek medical treatment at no cost and have the ability to see a medical specialist whenever necessary. He did state that he had no coverage for prescriptions. This young man lived in a remote area of western Canada and stated that he could easily get an appointment to see his physician whenever necessary. He was uncertain if this would be true in more densely populated areas of Canada.

According to the Pacific Research Institute, Canada ranks 24th out of 28 developed nations in doctors per 1000 people. This source also cited that approximately 825,000 Canadians were on waiting lists for surgery and other necessary treatments. In Great Britain, those awaiting surgery or hospital admission appear to be closer to one million. A study in the Lancet, a British medical journal compared survival rates for the top common cancers in the United States, Canada and Great Britain. The study concluded that Americans had a higher five-year survival rate over the other countries.

I personally believe socialized medicine is not the answer. If we look at socialized medicine in Europe, Canada and Australia, it appears that socialized medicine is more economical, but one must consider the trade off in the quality and expediency of care. Drawbacks include long waiting lists to see a physician, physician shortages and limited treatment options. Perhaps if we had more national private insurance companies the coverage costs for the insurers would be less. The idea should be entertained to pay for your own health insurance policy, similar to your homeowner's policy, and making health insurance portable to any state or job in which you live and work.

Chapter 6

WHEN THINGS GO AWRY

"Each patient ought to feel somewhat the better after the physician's visit, irrespective of the nature of the illness." ~Warfield Theobald Longcope

I understand that not everyone lives in a part of the country where physicians are plentiful or where their insurance coverage will cover second opinions. If you are in a situation that you are uncomfortable with a physician's plan of care, you should never hesitate to get another opinion. A confident doctor should not be threatened by your insistence for another opinion. Several years ago, I had gynecological surgery with a surgeon with whom I had worked for 15 years. He was a colleague of a physician that I completely trusted and respected. After my surgery, I had some disturbing symptoms that would not go away. At my postoperative office visit I discussed these issues on two occasions and my surgeon shrugged his shoulders and stated that what I was experiencing "happened sometimes." I even asked if I should consult a specialist and was told that I should wait six months to see if the symptoms disappeared. I didn't wait, I went to another gynecologist who not associated with the hospital in which I worked. I also requested a copy of my operative report. The operative report contains detailed information about what occurred during a surgical procedure. To my surprise, I read in the report that the surgeon had accidentally perforated my uterus during the surgery. It was repaired, but as a specialist told me later, sometimes the bladder becomes sutured to the uterus when the perforation is repaired. I was very upset at this information to put it mildly. I understand that medicine and surgery are not without errors. I did, however, have an issue with the fact that the surgeon never told me in the recovery room or in his office several weeks later what had occurred in the surgery. I never went back to that physician and never let him know that I found out. I continued to have problems for several months as a result of the surgery. I would have appreciated an explanation at the time of the incident so that I could better understand what my body was experiencing at that time.

My own mother's path to her death began when she was admitted to the hospital in November 2005 for a minor heart irregularity. The heart rhythm that she had at the time, atrial fibrillation, can lead to blood clots. Subsequently, she was given a drug called Coumadin, which is a well-known blood thinner. She had been on it years before, experienced some bleeding problems and was very reluctant to take it again. She had also been seeing a hematologist for several years for an unnamed bleeding disorder. I advised all the treating physicians of this information and asked that the hematologist be called in for a consultation as he had an office within the same hospital. Physician after physician told her it was safe and given routinely to patients with atrial fibrillation. Unfortunately, when my mother was transferred within the hospital and the orders were re-written by a physician, she was given 10 times the amount of Coumadin that she should have been prescribed, for a total of three days. I was never told by anyone at the hospital that this error had occurred. I had been away for the weekend and found her bleeding from all body openings upon my return. I made sure to inform the nurses and asked on more than one occasion that the physician be called. The nurses simply attributed bleeding from her nose as dryness from oxygen being given through her nose. Not satisfied, I closely examined my mother specifically where she said her leg had been hurting for 36 hours. Imagine my shock to see that all the skin on her lower leg had turned black. She had developed Coumadin-induced tissue necroses, a complication only experienced in less than 1 % of the patients that take Coumadin. Of course it was then a medical emergency that resulted in six weeks in the hospital and an additional six weeks in a rehabilitation facility to learn how to walk again after extensive skin grafts. After one of her skin graft surgeries, she woke up from surgery and could not move her finger. Her finger tendon had been overstretched and torn when she was on the operating room table. Of course the hospital wanted to disavow all knowledge and have her discharged and come back another time to fix her finger, which required more surgery. We insisted on the surgical repair during the same hospital stay and it was done. She did go to a rehabilitation facility, only to contract MRSA (Methicillin Resistant Staphylococcus Aureus.) This bacterial infection has been around for decades but has been in the news a lot more recently. It is a bacterial infection that seems to be more prevalent in hospitals and nursing homes, and once contracted, is difficult to treat.

It wasn't until a year after my mother's death, while reading her medical chart, that I found out about the amount of Coumadin that had been over-prescribed in the hospital. The ordering physician had made an error when reordering the medication. I was told that she was in urgent need of surgery to repair her leg but it could not be done at that time because laboratory reports indicated a dangerously elevated bleeding time. I was not informed then or at any other time during her hospital stay that it was due to a prescription error. She was in very critical condition and in danger of bleeding to death. No lawsuit was ever filed. An attorney informed me that it would be impossible to prove if the subsequent injury to the leg tissue would have developed on 1 mg as opposed to the 10 mg that was ordered in error.

Medical mishaps can occur any place and any time. Some are omissions of treatment. My sister-in-law was 50 years old when she died in 2006. She had been complaining to her personal care physician that her shoulder and arm were hurting for months. As the pain progressed, her physician told her it might be Lyme disease. She was given antibiotics that did nothing to ease the pain. She called the physician's office every few days to report her pain progression and was repeatedly told to "continue the antibiotics until they were all gone" - for a total of 20 days. The pain progressed and she was told she had either tendonitis or bursitis. She went to the local hospital emergency room and told the physician on duty, "I am here for a second opinion." The physician on duty never even examined her, but stated that they don't give second opinions and sent her on her way. Interestingly enough, she later requested her medical records pertaining to that Emergency Room visit. The same physician wrote that her exam was "normal" and yet several days later, she had a diagnosis of metastatic bone cancer! Prior to her diagnosis, her personal physician sent her for physical therapy. An astute physical therapist felt there was something else going on and suggested an MRI (Magnetic Resonance Imagining) was necessary. Of course, a physician needs to order an MRI. Her arm became progressively numb, and became paralyzed shortly thereafter. She called her personal physician and stated that she was going to the hospital and wanted an MRI done. The doctor told her to come immediately to the office, which she did. After a quick examination, she was told to go up to another floor of the doctor's office to see a neurologist. The neurologist picked up her arm - a very painful movement for her at the time - and forcefully pushed it down. My sister-in-law heard a loud crack and was in severe pain. She sat and cried until she could get enough energy to leave. An order was written for an MRI. Within hours, a diagnosis of metastatic bone cancer and a fracture, possibly induced by the neurologist when he forcefully pushed the already fragile, cancer-ridden bone. She bravely fought the cancer for a year until she lost the battle. Another lawsuit you may ask yourself? No, according to an attorney, in order to file an omission of cancer diagnosis lawsuit, the doctor must have misdiagnosed the cancer for a period of over one year. A woman that I know has duel degrees, in nursing and in law. She told me that mistakes made are not automatically grounds for a lawsuit. There has to be gross error or intent.

Another relative was also undiagnosed and poorly managed after a near drowning and spinal cord injury that would affect the rest of his life. This vibrant, healthy young man, dove headfirst into water and came up to the surface floating. CPR (cardiopulmonary resuscitation) was performed at the scene by friends and he was taken to a small community hospital without a backboard to immobilize his neck. He was unconscious the entire time. His stomach was pumped to empty the contents. It wasn't until about three hours later that an X-ray of this young man's neck was done only to discover that his neck had been broken and he would need to be transferred to a larger hospital. His immediate needs of neck immobilization and additional oxygen were not addressed adequately at the time of the emergency. The first neurosurgeon at the larger hospital advised letting this young man die, and did not want to stabilize or repair the neck fracture. Another neurosurgeon was located at the insistence of the family and took over his care. Today, he is a wonderful young man who now uses a wheelchair and is taking college courses. Sadly, we will never know what could have been if the initial care that he received was more attuned to his injury.

Most times you will not be informed if there was an error in your care. Hospital staff are required to fill out "incident reports" detailing what omissions or errors were made. But these are internal documents that do not make it onto the chart or become part of the medical record. Meetings are held behind closed doors to review serious health or death issues so that they can be evaluated by staff and prevented in the future.

A relative was told that it was likely that she had a cancerous tumor in her pancreas. She was advised to have immediate surgery. She opted to wait and go for a second opinion in a larger hospital.

She asked a family member to research surgeons and one was identified with many years of experience, having graduated from a top, well-known medical school. When she went for her visit, she stated the surgeon appeared somewhat pompous and kept telling her that he was the "Whipple King" (Whipple procedure is an operative procedure on the pancreas). He also told her that she did not have cancer, nor did she need surgery. She went back to her original gastroenterologist who sent her back to the larger hospital, to a surgeon who was a partner of the "Whipple King." She did have her surgery and it was cancerous. Fortunately, it was all self-contained and had not spread.

One man I know went to his urologist for recurrent symptoms. The physician said, "We'll do another PSA." (Prostate Specific Antigen is a blood test. An elevated level may indicate prostate cancer.) The patient replied that he had never had one done before. The physician stated, "Oh yes, you did." The physician had forgotten to order it previously, but ordered one at this visit. It came back high and the patient did in fact have prostate cancer. He had surgery at a large metropolitan cancer center and fortunately, his cancer had not spread.

Another man took his wife for a mammogram. She has advanced Alzheimer's and when it came time to do the test, she was taken into the testing room by her husband but ultimately she was too frightened to have it done. A week later, her husband got a report in the mail that the exam was normal. I have to wonder if her insurance got billed for the mammogram that was never done.

Here in Connecticut, a major hospital was cited by the State Department of Public Health for serious health violations, including four deaths: a baby died during labor, a man died due to a drug interaction, a man died in the emergency room while being evaluated for congestive heart failure and a woman who sought help for suicidal thoughts and was discharged, committed suicide three days later. (8) The hospital was to remain on probation for a year, in which time they will hire a clinical care consultant to evaluate their practices, modify them and attempt to improve on patient outcomes.

In October 2008, Healthcare Finance News reported that Yale-New Haven Hospital was fined $8,000 by the Connecticut Department of Public Health for failing to inspect patients for bedsores, administering wrong doses of medications and holding a patient against her will, which were all noted on unannounced inspections between August 2007 through March 2008.

Hospitals and nursing homes are also one of the most notorious places to pick up a deadly infection. According to the Centers for Disease Control, approximately 90,000 people die annually in the United States due to a hospital acquired infection.

One of the most important ways to avoid an infection is to require that every one that comes in contact with you wash their hands. This in itself may not be enough to prevent you from contracting MRSA, (methicillin-resistant staphylococcus aureus), a well known antibiotic resistant infection. Have nurses and physicians wash the end of the stethoscope with alcohol swabs prior to using it on you. In the hospital, wipe down telephones, television remotes, over bed trays and doorknobs in your room and bathroom. If a staff is unwilling to clean your environment and you are unable, enlist a family member to do it for you. Do not put personal belongings on the floor or use personal items or objects that have fallen onto the hospital floor. Get up and get moving as soon as your physician allows it. Do not let anyone touch your open wound or incision without clean gloves on. Don't be afraid to speak up. I have witnessed surgeons who have the best aseptic technique in the operating room get careless in the recovery phase of the patient. Unfortunately, this can have dire results.

Serious hospital, nursing home or home health agency errors, omissions or neglect should be reported to the Joint Commission (JACHO). This can be accomplished by a phone call, anonymous letter or e-mail. You should not report billing issues, insurance or personnel issues to the Joint Commission. Contact information for the Joint Commission is in the Resources Information section of the book.

PHARMACEUTICAL MISTAKES

According to a National Academies report issued in 2006, it is estimated that there are well over 7,000 deaths per year in the United States attributed to pharmaceutical mistakes. These occurrences can be the wrong medication, the wrong dose, the wrong prescription or the wrong combination of medications. Many may never be recognized for what they are or reported as such, so these numbers may be underreported.

Prescription mistakes can occur at any time and anywhere. The physician may order the wrong dose, the pharmacist may interpret the prescription incorrectly or the patient may take the wrong dosage. There are many variables when dealing with pharmaceutical errors.

Pharmacists are human and make errors also. Pharmacy mistakes can occur within or outside of a hospital setting. Some pharmacies are extremely busy, with multiple distractions and although they do not intentionally give out the wrong prescription, it does happen.

You should be familiar with your medication and dosages and not be afraid to question any medication that does not look right. Your pharmacist is an excellent resource person regarding your medication. His time and advice is free. He can advise you regarding interactions with your current medications, side effects and actions. Few people take the time to really understand their medication or the implications and consequences of taking it incorrectly.

I have witnessed many errors at a national chain pharmacy in my town. They were dispensing prescriptions to the wrong customers: they had the correct last name but neglected to verify the patients' first name.

I picked up a prescription for my mother and it was double her usual dose of a "water" pill. I knew the correct dosage and read the label when I got home. I double checked it and recognized the error before giving my mother the pill. I returned to the pharmacy to notify them of the error. The pharmacy refunded the money, filled it correctly for free, and apologized.

When talking to other family members, I heard several more stories of errors at the same pharmacy. My aunt was given a thyroid medication that was prescribed for someone with the same last name. She thought it was the antibiotic that her doctor had ordered, as she did not notice the first name on the label was not hers. She took the thyroid pill and called her doctor and the pharmacy when she noticed the mistake. Luckily, she suffered no adverse effects.

Be sure to read the accompanying papers that come with a prescription. It will give you a brief description of the medication, its uses and side effects. If it does not sound like something your doctor ordered, check with the pharmacy or the ordering physician before taking it.

Another family member used the same pharmacy in our town. She was taking an antibiotic for an infection. By the third day, she was familiar with the pills in the bottle. On the fourth day, she noted a pill that was a different size, shape and color from the same bottle. She immediately went to the pharmacy to ascertain what had happened. Apparently, the pharmacy ran out of one antibiotic and substituted another without telling the patient.

When all of these issues came to light, I looked to a state agency to notify of these errors. I found a phone number and made a call to the Division of Drug Control at the Connecticut Department of Consumer Protection. The state representative said they had no record of other errors at this pharmacy. I thought this was peculiar because I had heard so many instances of errors there. When I checked back with others, I learned they had never reported the errors to the state, but felt it was the pharmacy's responsibility to inform the state of their own errors. I was informed by the state that the pharmacy that makes the error is responsible for policing itself. In other words, the pharmacy likes to handle their errors internally. The errors do not get reported to a state agency unless the patient makes the call. But most people will not make the call. They will return the medication where the pharmacy will do their best to "make it right," usually at no cost to the patient. This means a pharmacy can continue what it had been doing with no repercussions.

So I went back to the pharmacy and watched quietly, as the pharmacists filled prescriptions, answered phones and rang up the register. I also noted that the prescriptions were being time stamped as they were taken out of a bin to be filled. When I asked the pharmacist, I was told that at this particular pharmacy, the staff is actually timed by upper management. I was told that slow work was a reason for a poor evaluation. That didn't sound like good practice for a pharmacy. I know we are all rushed, but I prefer to have my pharmacist take an extra minute to be sure he has the right drug for the right person. Of interest, I had stopped going to that particular pharmacy myself years ago, but my mother did not have a prescription plan and continued to go there. She had priced her prescriptions at several area pharmacies and felt that one had the best prices. I had also personally noted a lot of the pharmacists leaving employment there over the years.

So unless you call your State Department of Consumer Protection, and report these errors, these mistakes are not documented - the pharmacy keeps this information to themselves. It appears that some corporate pharmacy chains care more about time and production - not accuracy. So let's all make the pharmacies accountable for accuracy and report errors to our State Department of Consumer Protection.

According to the U.S. Pharmacopeia Convention, a nonprofit drug standard-setting group, there are nearly 3,200 prescription medications with names that sound or look alike. (9) Another man that I know was given a wrong prescription at a pharmacy TWICE! Instead of a thyroid medication, he was given a medication for cancer. The names of these drugs were reportedly very similar.

You may possibly avoid this type of error by asking the prescribing physician the name and type of medication when it is initially ordered. Ask the pharmacist the same questions and the answers should be similar. If one answers that it is for heartburn and the other answers that it is used for anxiety, at least you will have a clue that there was miscommunication along the way and resolve to get the answers prior to taking the medication.

No one is immune to medication errors. Recently, twin newborn children of actor Dennis Quaid and his wife were given accidental overdoses of the drug heparin while in a California hospital. The labels of the medication vials reportedly "looked similar." The drug company is now looking into changing the labels so this error is less likely to be repeated in the future.

A television news investigation in my home state also addressed this topic in July 2002, stating that pharmacy errors are on the rise.

A Team Eight (a local television station in Connecticut), investigation has discovered an alarming increase in the number of errors at pharmacies in Connecticut.

The numbers are startling. According to the Division of Drug Control at the Connecticut Department of Consumer Protection, the number of investigated and confirmed pharmacy errors has steadily risen from 8 in 1987 to 30 in 1995, 61 in 1998, and 91 in 2001 and in the first half of 2002 there were 73 confirmed errors at pharmacies across the state. In the most recent data available, an attorney who investigates pharmacy errors reported there were 92 investigated and confirmed pharmacy errors in Connecticut in 2006.

A retired pharmacist, who spent 32 years in the industry, said in the news report, "We filled 250 prescriptions in 660 minutes. That comes out to 2.6 minutes that you're allowed to devote to counseling, filling a prescription and getting it out to a patient. Dangerous, very dangerous."

Why are pharmacists so overworked? There is a nationwide shortage of pharmacists. That comes as the number of prescriptions is exploding. From 2.5 billion across the country in 2001 to over four billion expected by 2005. (10)

Pharmacists also must spend a large amount of time counseling consumers, dealing with insurance companies, managed care companies and HMOs.

What you can do -

At Home:

- Make a list of your prescribed medications. Include any vitamin supplements that you take.
- Bring your medication list with you to all your doctor appointments for review.
- Be informed about your medications; read about them. The Physicians Desk Reference is the gold standard for medications. Your local library should have a current book. However, your pharmacy may have a smaller book available on prescriptions that is easier to understand.
- Read the literature that comes with the prescribed medication. It will list uses, side effects and possible other dangerous medication and food combinations.
- If you cannot take a medication or continue it, notify your physician.

At the Pharmacy:

- Read the label while you are still at the pharmacy. Make sure you know what medicine you are picking up and how it is to be used. This information should coincide with information your physician told you.

- Ask for written information regarding your prescription.
- Clarify any possible interactions or side effects with the pharmacist and/or your physician.

In the Hospital:

- Make sure the person administering your medication is checking your identity each time they bring medication to you. The Joint Commission recommends two identity checks at each visit, asking you to state your name and checking your identification bracelet. Some hospitals now have bar code scanners and will scan your identity bracelet prior to administering medication.
- Ask for a printed sheet of the medication you will be receiving. Keep the list at your bedside and reference it each time a medication is taken. Many modern hospitals have electronic records and a medication sheet can be printed in seconds.
- Find out the purpose or expected effect of the medication.
- Ask the name of the medication and dosage each and every time it is brought to you.
- Note the appearance of the medication that you are taking, such as the size and color of the pills.

Changes are being discussed and implemented daily to ensure that the correct medications are prescribed for the correct patient.

Senators John Kerry (D. Massachusetts), and Newt Gingrich, former speaker of the House and founder of the Center for Health Transformation, wrote in a Wall Street Journal article that they supported the switch to electronic prescriptions. They conclude, "E-prescribing for Medicare is just the beginning of the modernization and digitization our ailing health care system urgently needs. A high-tech, healthier future is within our grasp," (Kerry/Gingrich, Wall Street Journal, 11/16). (11) Supporters of this system conclude that fewer transcription errors will be made. They also conclude an electronic copy of your prescription allows for easier access in case of a national disaster or the need to refill while traveling out of state.

The FDA (United States Food and Drug Administration) is entrusted to ensure the quality of our food supply, vitamin and dietary supplements, medications and medical products are safe. They also report on false advertising, false health products, harm from medical products and prescriptions. Their Web site contains various reports and warning letters to drug companies regarding actual cited violations and/or their lack of documentation. This in itself is concerning as many Americans need their medication to survive and we rely on the drug companies to provide us with the

71

proper drug and the proper dosage in a hygienic, uncontaminated manner. Furthermore, we expect that the Food and Drug Administration will be standing over their shoulder making sure that the drug companies are in compliance. However, errors continue to be made to this day.

On the FDA Web site you can research recalled medications and even sign up for automatic e-mail alerts from MedWatch. Any time the FDA posts a new warning about a suspected dangerous medication, nutritional supplement or medical equipment or device, you will automatically be alerted by e-mail. You can also submit adverse reactions to any medication or medical device online at the FDA Web site. See back of book under Resources Information for Web site addresses. If you prefer you can check the Web site often, to view medication and equipment recalls as soon as the FDA issues them.

Some prescription horror stories have surfaced regarding the manufacturing process of medications. In 2006, a major United States drug manufacturer of acetaminophen had to pull it off the store shelves due to metal fragments found within the pills. The mishap was due to deteriorating machinery used in the manufacture of acetaminophen - more commonly known as Tylenol.

Likewise, many American based companies have moved their manufacturing plants to foreign countries in order to save on manufacturing and labor costs. Many of the large drug companies that we associate with being "American" are physically located in Puerto Rico, a commonwealth of the United States. Twenty of the best selling United States prescriptions are manufactured in Puerto Rico. In February 2008, a worker at one of the drug manufacturing plants in Puerto Rico noted blue colored flecks of paint on medications. The blue flecks were later determined to be the same blue paint that was on the building's doors. The FDA refused to step in, citing the incident as "isolated." The Canadian company that owns the manufacturing plant did nothing to stop the shipment of the medication to the United States or to determine how widespread the problem was. (12) Allegations of inaccurate dosing and manufacturing contamination continue to surround popular medications produced in the Caribbean, China and India, and used in the United States today.

In February 2008, Baxter International, a large U.S. pharmaceutical company, was involved in an investigation regarding its production of heparin in its China facility. Production of heparin was suspended after many patients experienced severe allergic reactions and some patients died. "As to the Chinese factory that has come to the U.S. regulators' attention, this is just another case of Chinese safety and quality standards being questioned, after health concerns were raised over the past years by imports such as toothpaste, toys, seafood and other food products." (13)

The FDA appears to be slow in its response to the issue of heparin contamination and allergic reactions. It wasn't until weeks later that the FDA issued a statement that it would test all heparin products prior to importing them into the United States. In March 2008, it was determined that Heparin manufactured in China was contaminated with oversulfated chondroitin sulfate which was responsible for the previous adverse reactions and deaths. Oversulfated chondroitin sulfate is a man-made chemical and the FDA is not reporting how it made its way into the heparin. (14)

In September 2008, the U.S. Government closed our borders to more than 30 generic drugs made by India's drug giant Ranbaxy Laboratories because of poor quality in two of its factories. Some of these drugs included popular antibiotics, cholesterol lowering medication and a medication used to control diabetes.

The list of medications that appears to have bypassed the scrutiny of the FDA continues to grow. Due to complaints of AIDS activists in the 1980's, the FDA responded by decreasing the length of time for approval for marketing new drugs. The length of time went from a median of 22 months in 1992 to less than 12 months in 1999, although a slight increase was seen for the year 2000. (15) Since the year 2000, more than a dozen drugs have been pulled off the market including such prescriptions as Fen-Phen, Vioxx, Celebrex and Bextra, which came under scrutiny for possibly causing serious side effects and even deaths. Some additional drugs that were pulled off the American market after release include, Rezulin, Lotronox and Baycol, while others simply got a "black box warning" label attached to identify possible health risks associated with these medications. The FDA's Center for Drug Evaluation and Research only approved 20 new medicines with new chemical compounds in 2005, and only 22 in 2006. So it appears that they are taking a little longer to investigate and approve new medications prior to releasing them to the public.

One solution for getting new drugs to market quicker was to hire more people at the FDA. To do that, more money was needed. So in 1992, The 1992 Prescription Drug User Fees Act was passed and the FDA was allowed to collect user fees from the pharmaceutical companies. These fees were in excess of 5 million dollars in the 2007 FDA budget. The FDA's 2008 fiscal year budget also projects increased user fees collected from pharmaceutical companies to allow for more inspections of the FDA approved drug manufacturing facilities, improving generic drug reviews and modernizing drug safety issues including communication. The 2008 proposed generic drug user fees were budgeted at over 15 million dollars. These are all positive responses to enable newer medications onto the market, thereby lowering the costs of brand name drugs.

So now, we have the pharmaceutical companies paying the FDA to approve their new medications. Some critics argue that this system of payment may influence the FDA to approve drugs that it had not previously. One of those critics is Dr. Sidney Wolfe.

According to Dr. Wolfe, Director of Public Citizen's Health Research Group, "in Washington, the pharmaceutical industry will give the FDA $150 million in cash directly from the industry to the FDA to run their drug review process. So, the whole process is corrupt, to say the very least; and the people that suffer are the American public. The drug industry, understandably, is trying to sell drugs, and the FDA doesn't bother very often to enforce the laws on false and misleading advertising; and so what people see on television, what doctors see in their office, with respect to the risks and benefits of drugs, are wrong. But the FDA is supposed to be representing the public. The FDA, though, getting money from the drug industry, is not putting out accurate information."

Dr. Wolfe has published a book, entitled, "Worst Pills, Best Pills, A Consumer's Guide to Avoiding Drug-Induced Death or Illness," in collaboration with Larry D. Sasich, Pharm D., M.P.H., and Rose Ellen Hope, R.Ph., Pocket Books, 1999, ISBN # 067101918X. He has referenced FDA files from published studies to come to his conclusions (16). In his book, he highlights many of the popular medications on the market and some of the potential benefits and adverse reactions to medications.

The same Dr. Wolfe testified before a House Subcommittee in February of 2008. He stated that the Food and Drug Administration is suffering from "a crisis in leadership, a lack of congressional oversight and a dangerous reliance on the pharmaceutical industry to bankroll it operations." He states the FDA is funded almost 2/3 by the drug industry. (17)

Insurance coverage and reimbursement for prescriptions seems to be a revolving dilemma. Insurance companies want to pay the least amount possible for a prescription. So if you choose to take one of the newer drugs just approved by the FDA, you must be cautious regarding any side effects and report them to your doctor immediately. Ask your doctor if he is sending written information regarding your adverse reaction to the appropriate agencies. You can also file a report yourself with the Food and Drug Administration either in writing or through their Web site. The decision to take a newer medication on the market has to be a decision based on a conversation between you and your physician.

Prescription drugs are a multi-billion dollar business. Pharmaceutical representatives are also visiting your physician's offices and hospitals, bringing lunch for the staff to promote new drug therapies. Sometimes physicians are treated to dinners and gifts by the pharmaceutical representatives. Some large medical schools are just beginning to ban these luncheons and gifts. The concern is that a physician may be influenced by gifts to prescribe a specific medication. A June 23, 2008 report by the Fraser Institute disputes this hypothesis by reporting that in 2007, 67% of all U.S. prescriptions were for generic medication and not brand name medication. That would suggest that the pharmaceutical representatives might not have as much control over prescription trends as previously thought.

A new grassroots movement is coming into play in some states to counteract the pharmaceutical representatives. Pennsylvania is one such state. State representatives are trying to facilitate effective medication treatment for their residents by educating physicians regarding the costs of generics. These states are paying for consultants, such as registered nurses and others, to go into physician offices, much like a pharmaceutical representative would, and encourage physicians to consider prescribing generics, less expensive medications and less expensive treatments which may include lifestyle changes. The goal is to hold down costs for some of the state-subsidized programs. Other states trying similar tactics are West Virginia, Vermont and South Carolina. (18)

Consumers and consumer advocates are also demanding more honesty in pharmaceutical advertising. A recent Lipitor television commercial was filmed and aired in Connecticut for a few months featuring Dr. Robert Jarvik. Similar commercials with Dr. Jarvik promoting Lipitor aired nationwide. As the sales of Lipitor increased dramatically after both newspaper and commercial advertisements, consumers complained that Dr. Jarvik, who was associated with the first "artificial heart" and was the spokesman for Lipitor, never completed his medical internship nor had he ever practiced medicine. The local television advertisement for Lipitor disappeared as quickly as it came. Other ads that featured Dr. Jarvik promoting Lipitor were criticized when it was discovered that Dr. Jarvik had used stunt doubles in some of the television ads. These television ads were also removed from the air.

In the past several years, there was an influx of television ads of men in white coats, wearing a stethoscope around their neck, pitching the sales and treatments for many pharmaceuticals. At the end of the commercial, in fine print, a disclaimer revealed that the man portraying a physician in the commercial was, in fact, an actor and not a physician. Then tactics seemed to switch to using celebrities to endorse specific medications. For a substantial fee, celebrities put their names and faces with pharmaceutical products. However, that advertising tactic seemed short lived and appears to be scarce today. Now, celebrities are being less obvious with their sales pitches and instead are promoting treatments for illnesses through awareness campaigns.

In many European countries, it is illegal to advertise prescription pharmaceuticals directly to consumers. This leaves more of the prescribing influence on the physician. Consumers are not bombarded with television, newspaper or magazine ads promoting the latest pharmaceuticals or even homeopathic products.

Any ads that are approved must be factual and not promoted as cure-alls or rejuvenation products.

My recommendation would be to talk to your physician about prescribing tried and true pharmaceuticals that have been on the market for several years, rather than the new ones that are just coming out. Dr. Sidney Wolfe advises waiting until a drug has been on the market for seven years to determine if it is safe. Educate yourself about the medications that you are taking and report any adverse or unexpected side effects to your physician immediately.

Ask your physician if you can start at the lowest dose possible until you determine if you have any adverse reactions to a new medication. Report any new symptoms to your physician after starting a new medication. They may be related. Ask your physician the intended duration of any new medication and follow his directions. Clarify all instructions with your physician prior to leaving the office.

I feel that I must add a word of caution here regarding prescription medications. I know from witnessing firsthand that many of my mother's generation will give their unused medications that they no longer need to their friends. Some may be on a similar medication and want to "save some money" and not waste what has already been purchased. This is never a good idea. Dosages may vary and a small change may be detrimental to a good friend's health. Some medications may also be less effective due to the age

80

and improper storage of the medication. Some can even become toxic over time. So it is never a good idea to pass on unused medication in any form to a friend or relative. A July 2008 article in the Archives of Internal Medicine, reported that fatal medication errors in the home environment increased greater than 360% in the years between 1983 and 2004. More people are dying from improper use of prescription medication than ever before. AARP (American Association of Retired Persons) has excellent information on their Web site regarding the safe use of prescription medication in addition to a personal medication record that can be downloaded and printed. See the Resources Information section in the back of this book.

Medication should be disposed of safely when no longer needed. Make sure that children or animals cannot get into the disposed medication. The correct way to dispose of unused medi-cation has come under question. Apparently, many of us have been flushing unused or outdated medications into our private and public septic systems for years as we were previously told. The con-tamination of our drinking water with trace amounts of medication has been highlighted in the news in 2008. The Environmental Protection Agency (EPA) apparently is just beginning to take this subject seriously. A statement on their Web site reports: "The EPA is committed to investigating this topic and developing strategies to help protect the health of both the environment and the public. To date, scientists have found no evidence of adverse human health effects from PPCPs in the environment."(19) The EPA currently does not require that public drinking water be tested for pharmaceutical elements. Through natural elimination, our medication travels through our bodies and into our septic or sewer system. Those with public sewers have their waste treated at waste treatment plants and eventually the treated water is released back into our rivers and streams. Testing of treated public city water across the nation has shown evidence of trace amounts of variable medications. The long-term effect of ingesting such trace amounts of medication is not known. Flushing medication down the toilet is not the best way to dispose of medication. A local pharmacist advised me to put unused, crushed and watered down medication into old coffee grounds, kitty litter or sawdust, adding water and sealing tightly so no animals or children could get the medication prior to putting it in the trash. Some municipal or local trash companies may have services available for incineration of these potentially toxic substances. Check with your local government or trash collector.

Some pharmacies have "clean out your medicine cabinet day" to allow you to collect and drop off your old medication for proper disposal for free. Check with your local pharmacy to see if they would be able to coordinate and assist in this endeavor. I checked with several local pharmacies in my area regarding this issue. None of them held collection days. One of three that I spoke with (Osco) would accept unused or unwanted prescriptions that would be discarded with their regular garbage. The pharmacist was unclear if any special precautions would be taken with the disposal. It is also unclear if this is a national policy with this pharmacy or would vary at each location.

Two other pharmacists that I spoke with in top national chains did not know of any group that would accept collections. They were both aware of the water contamination issue of prescription medications in drinking water. Both advised not flushing unused medication. One pharmacist advised putting all unused medication in one container and adding enough water to dilute the medications to make them unusable and then throwing them in the household garbage.

There are some agencies that will accept donated medications. The Star Fish Project, associated with New York Presbyterian Hospital, will accept some types of medications. They will provide a Federal Express shipping label at no charge for those who want to send medication. The medication must be in its original container with the prescription label affixed. The medication must not be outdated. It is sent to foreign countries for those who cannot get medication by other means and the label is removed prior to shipping out of the country. For those interested in donating, the Star Fish Project information is located in the back of this book under the heading of "Resources Information." Currently, it is illegal to redistribute medication that has left the hands of the distributor in the United States. It can legally be given to other countries as "humanitarian aid." The State of Missouri has a donation program run by the Department of Health and Senior Services. Check with your state to see if there is such a program in place. (Please note that there are many United States agencies that will accept used canes, wheelchairs, walkers and other medical equipment. Please check with your local VNA, nursing home or social service agency for recommendations and suggestions.)

The topic of safe disposal of unused medication is just beginning to come to the forefront. I think as time goes on, we will see more information on this important issue. In Connecticut, there are currently no regulatory changes regarding medication disposal, however, the Department of Public Health and the Department of Environmental Protection are promoting an educational public awareness campaign.

In regards to medication advice, I was told a disturbing story in the spring of 2008. A trusted family friend advised a long-term seizure patient that he needed to stop his anti-seizure medication - "that stuff can be really bad for you." Ill advised, the person did just that and within a month suffered a grandmal seizure. Fortunately, there were no serious injuries in this instance, but for this young man, confined to a wheelchair with a spinal cord injury, the consequences could have been disastrous. The well-meaning friend did not intend harm, but did not understand the realm of the person's health history and implications of foregoing medication. It is never wise to give prescription medication advice to or take it from someone other than your physician or pharmacist.

Another area to be cautious about is the popular practice of using naturopathic medications, vitamins and herbal supplements. These remedies have been used for centuries by ancient cultures. However, you need to know that the Food and Drug Administration does not supervise the manufacture or import of such products from foreign countries. The amount and purity of these remedies may vary greatly with each distributor. Some of the more popular natural herbal remedies include ginseng, garlic, echinacea, chamomile, ginkgo biloba, saw palmetto, fever few, black cohosh and St. John's wort. Just because a product is labeled "natural" does not mean that it is safe for everyone. There are many of herbal medications on the market. Your local library or naturopathic doctors are good sources of information on naturopathic medications. Choose a state licensed practitioner or one that is certified by a leading naturopathic organization. A naturopathic doctor (N.D.), is a general practitioner that believes the body has the ability to heal itself naturally. The focus may be on treating underlying causes of an illness and treating the whole person. Ask this practitioner how much experience they have had treating a symptom or illness similar to yours. Generally, alternative medication is used to complement your traditional medication, not replace it. Make sure that all treating practitioners are aware of all the treatments and prescriptions that you are taking, especially herbals. If you do decide to take naturopathic medications you should look for a "USP (United States Pharmacopoeia) verified" mark on the label. This verification ensures the consumer that this product has been tested for quality, strength and purity and has met the standards of the United States Pharmacopoeia. Also consult with your personal physician prior to starting a naturopathic regimen and again if your experience a change in your health status. Your physician needs to know which of these products you are taking and in what amounts. Some of them may interact with your prescribed medication and render it useless or even dangerous. Be sure to carry a list of ALL forms of medication that you are taking. Bring the original pills in their original containers to your physician. Ask your physician and pharmacist to review your medications each time a new one is added. Review which ones are necessary to continue and which ones need to be stopped when a new one is added.

Other practitioners that treat illness and injury with a de-emphasis on prescription medication are chiropractors, acupuncturists, massage therapists and biofeedback specialists. Chiropractors focus on drug-free, hands-on approach to treating muscle and bone problems, inflammation, pain and decreased range of motion by the manipulation and adjustment of joints. Many chiropractor treatments are covered under medical health care plans although the fees and coverage may vary.

Acupuncture is the insertion of thin needles into specific body points by either an acupuncturist or trained anesthesiologist. It is now being administered in many pain centers across the United States by anesthesiologists and may be covered by insurance. There are many freestanding facilities that also offer acupuncture by trained acupuncturists and your insurance may be less likely to cover treatment in one of these facilities. Do make sure that any facility you visit for acupuncture treatment is inspected and regulated by the state in which you live.

Massage therapy can also be used as an alternative to prescription medication. Massage is the application of pressure to muscle and soft tissue to promote circulation and reduce tension and pain. Massage therapy performed in a physical therapy office may be covered by health insurance when prescribed by a physician but not covered when performed in a day spa.

Biofeedback uses relaxation and visualization techniques to re-train the mind to control such body sensors such as breathing, heart rate, skin temperature and muscle tension. Biofeedback may or may not be covered by your health insurance provider.

Some possible beneficial supplements you may want to discuss with your physician include the use of daily low dose aspirin, fish oil tablets, calcium and vitamin D.

If you don't believe that pharmaceuticals are a big business, consider this. According to Forbes.com, in 2005, Miles D. White the CEO of Abbott Laboratories, a large U.S. pharmaceutical company, had been compensated with 26.2 million dollars worth of company stock shares in addition to his 1.61 million dollar annual salary and 2.65 million dollar bonus. (20)

Chapter 7

DOCUMENT, DOCUMENT, DOCUMENT

"Documentation is like sex: when it is good, it is very, very good; and when it is bad, it is better than nothing" - Dick Brandon

Nursing has helped me in many aspects of my life. One of the cardinal rules in nursing school was, "If you didn't chart it, it didn't happen." I have transferred that knowledge to everyday issues in my life. When I have phone conversations with insurance companies, utility companies or have other important interactions, I make a note of the time and date and ask for a name and call back number. Some companies will also give you an "incident number" if you ask. This will allow you a quick reference number if you should need to call back regarding the same issue. I keep files with the pertinent paperwork and it has helped me time and time again.

So what does this have to do with you and your doctor? Keep a journal, note pad or computer program with a list of your doctor visits, chief complaints, doctor recommendations, tests, test results, medications and any other pertinent information. Revise it after each interaction with your doctor. After days, weeks and years, it is difficult to remember the who, what, where and when of your medical care. You will have it all at your fingertips.

- Keep a medical journal on yourself and immediate family.
- Include your physician's name, address and phone number.
- Include any allergies to food or medication that you may have.
- Include an emergency contact list with phone numbers.
- Keep a comprehensive list of your medications, dosages and scheduling.
- Note any medical tests done - date and location - and relevant information, such as test results.
- Bring this to all physician appointments, medical tests and hospital visits.

By documenting your care and physician visits in the hospital, you may also uncover billing mistakes. These can be difficult to prove, but a detailed journal can provide clues to charges that are included on your hospital bill for items that were never received or testing or treatment that was not done. Hospital billing errors do occur and can be expensive if you are the one paying the bill.

Chapter 8

MEDICAL BILLING ERRORS

"My doctor game me six months to live, but when I couldn't pay the bill he gave me six months more." - Walter Matthau

Anyone who has been hospitalized or has other concerns regarding their medical bills, should request an itemized bill be sent to them in writing. It is estimated that thousands of errors go undetected every year and are simply paid by the insurance provider.

Many hospital charges are entered into the system and never removed if the procedure or test is canceled. This is when a written log at your bedside can come in handy or into use to verify your inpatient hospital bill. Each day a physician enters your hospital room, a charge is incurred for the visit. Write down each visit and by what specialist.

The Medical Billing Advocates of America, (MBAA), maintains a Web site for those who need assistance with their hospital or medical billing concerns. Pat Palmer formed MBAA in

1997 after working for a health insurance company for years. After seeing thousands of billing errors, she chose to become a consumer advocate in the field of medical billing errors. Some outrageous examples of medical billing on their Web site include:

- A trip to the emergency room cost one couple in Georgia $40,000.
- A box of tissues, which costs about $ 2.00 was billed as a "mucus recovery system" for the amount of $12.00.
- A baby girl was billed for a circumcision.
- A 2x2 piece of gauze used to wipe down surgical equipment, was billed for $57.00 as a "fog elimination device."
- A hospital gave a patient a toothbrush as a courtesy-- and then charged her $1,004 for it. (21)

Medicare and other health insurance providers are now stepping forward and denying coverage for extra costs associated with preventable hospital errors or conditions that develop in hospitalized patients. Some of these include falls from a hospital bed, bedsores and/or infections that were acquired in the hospital. The coverage for urinary tract infections that were acquired during the hospital stay has been targeted for non-coverage. At the present time, there is no standard for waiving hospital fees for such errors, but reviews and allowances are made on a case-by-case basis.

By creating a national standard, hospitals will be accountable for a higher standard of care and be ultimately responsible financially when criteria are not met.

The National Quality Forum has come up with a list of 28 events that should NEVER occur in the health setting. These are referred to as "Never Events."

As defined by the National Quality Forum, they are:

- Artificial insemination with the wrong donor sperm or donor egg.
- Unintended retention of a foreign object in a patient after surgery or other procedure.
- Patient death or serious disability associated with patient elopement (disappearance).
- Patient death or serious disability associated with a medication error (e.g., errors involving the wrong drug, wrong dose, wrong patient, wrong time, wrong rate, wrong preparation or wrong route of administration).
- Patient death or serious disability associated with a hemolytic reaction due to the administration of ABO/HLA-incompatible blood or blood products.

• Patient death or serious disability associated with an electric shock or elective cardioversion while being cared for in a healthcare facility.

• Patient death or serious disability associated with a fall while being cared for in a healthcare facility.

• Surgery performed on the wrong body part.

• Surgery performed on the wrong patient.

• Wrong surgical procedure performed on a patient.

• Intra-operative or immediately postoperative death in an ASA Class I patient. (The ASA classification is a standardized rating used by the American Society of Anesthesiologists. It rates the overall assessed health of a patient who is to undergo anesthesia. A Class I patient is a "normal healthy patient.")

• Patient death or serious disability associated with the use of contaminated drugs, devices or biologics provided by the healthcare facility.

• Patient death or serious disability associated with the use or function of a device in patient care, in which the device is used or functions other than as intended.

• Patient death or serious disability associated with intravascular air embolism that occurs while being cared for in a healthcare facility.

• Infant discharged to the wrong person.

• Patient suicide, or attempted suicide resulting in serious disability, while being cared for in a healthcare facility.

• Maternal death or serious disability associated with labor or delivery in a low-risk pregnancy while being cared for in a healthcare facility.

• Patient death or serious disability associated with hypoglycemia, the onset of which occurs while the patient is being cared for in a healthcare facility.

• Death or serious disability (kernicterus) associated with failure to identify and treat hyperbilirubinemia in neonates.

• Stage 3 or 4 pressure ulcers acquired after admission to a healthcare facility.

• Patient death or serious disability due to spinal manipulative therapy.

• Any incident in which a line designated for oxygen or other gas to be delivered to a patient contains the wrong gas or is contaminated by toxic substances.

• Patient death or serious disability associated with a burn incurred from any source while being cared for in a healthcare facility.

• Patient death or serious disability associated with the use of restraints or bed rails while being cared for in a healthcare facility.

• Any instance of care ordered by or provided by someone impersonating a physician, nurse, pharmacist, or other licensed healthcare provider.

• Abduction of a patient of any age.

• Sexual assault on a patient within or on the grounds of the healthcare facility.

• Death or significant injury of a patient or staff member resulting from a physical assault (i.e., battery) that occurs within or on the grounds of the healthcare facility" (22)

Currently, 39 states still bill the patient or the insurance provider for medical errors such as those on the "Never Events" list. Some states have chosen to pick and chose which "Never Events" are billable and which are not.

You will need to check with your state regarding laws affecting billing for medical mistakes. The trends are changing toward making hospitals more liable for paying for their own errors.

According to the U.S. Centers for Medicare and Medicaid Services after October 1, 2008, they no longer reimburse hospitals for the following "preventable" conditions and complications:

•   catheter-associated urinary tract infections.

•   stage III or IV pressure ulcers.

•   air embolism.

- falls and trauma resulting in fractures.
- burns or serious injuries.
- blood incompatibility.
- mediastinitis after coronary artery bypass graft (a surgical site infection.)

In addition to the above list, and additional 8 - 14 conditions and complications are under consideration for nonpayment through Medicare.

In some cases, patients have even been billed for medical mistakes. For example, a patient was scheduled for hernia repair surgery in Iowa, mistakenly was operated on the wrong side before the surgeon noted his error and performed the surgery on the correct side during the same surgery. The patient's health insurance provider was billed for both operations. (23)

Always ask for an itemized hospital bill and be sure to review it carefully. If you kept a journal during your hospitalization, it may help you review the charges for discrepancies.

Chapter 9

THE GOOD, THE BAD AND THE UGLY

"Never go to a doctor whose office plants have died." - Erma
Bombeck

As I discussed previously, there are many wonderful,
talented, skilled and compassionate people working in the field of
medicine. There are also a handful that are mentally ill themselves
or are addicts of some sort.

In my home state of Connecticut, a case came to light
regarding a deceased endocrinologist. His previous home had been
sold and the new owners knocked out a wall in a basement to find
thousands of pictures of child pornography. These pictures are
reportedly photos taken by the physician of his patients who were
children - many photos taken with the parents' knowledge and
permission, but for the physician's own use. It appears that they
were not taken for medical reasons due to the fact that he had hidden
them in a concealed room in his basement. As of mid-January,

2008, 59 people were suing the hospital where the physician practiced. (24). This number is only a fraction of the actual pictures that were found and of the people that had come forward at that time. It is a sad reminder that we all need to be vigilant. When our young children, friends or family are in the healthcare system, we need to keep our eyes and ears open. I have known a few people that felt that they were either touched inappropriately or viewed unnecessarily by a physician. In one instance, one medical resident was asked to leave the training program soon after the incident was relayed to a senior physician by a patient. Two other practicing physicians continued practicing - with no formal complaints against them - however, both patients did not go back to the respective physicians. Young children, the elderly and mentally challenged may not be able to speak up or know when something is inappropriate. They need an advocate who has their best interest in mind and will ensure their safety. If a physician will not allow a family member or friend in an exam or procedure room, ask that another licensed professional or staff member be present if the situation warrants it. For example, a male physician performing an examination on a female patient should have a female medical assistant in the room with him. Not only does this protect the patient, but also the physician from any false accusations from patients. If the physician will not honor this request, it should at the very least, raise some suspicions. However, if you and your physician have a long-standing professional relationship and you are comfortable and the physician is comfortable with no "chaperone," it should be up to the physician's discretion.

Medicine is not an exact science. It is the practice of one or more medical professionals using their scientific knowledge and experience to attempt to determine the cause of a sign or symptom.

If medical mistakes counted among the leading causes of death in America, they would be eighth. A report issued by the Institute of Medicine estimated at least 44,000 and perhaps as many as 98,000 hospitalized Americans die every year from medical errors. (25).

Mistakes are easily made and sometimes a process of elimination has to be utilized to sort out the real issue. Valuable time and money can be lost during this process and it is critical for the patient to be as honest and accurate as possible when describing their symptoms. This is not always the case. Sometimes the "blame" falls to the patient. A dear friend of mine, a retired nurse, often accompanies her family members to the doctor. Time after time, she is frustrated when the "patient" gets into the exam room and tells the doctor that everything is fine and minimizes or just fails to mention what the real problem is. Sometimes, the patient will just talk about issues not related to medicine or symptoms altogether. She deals with this by talking on the phone to the doctors whenever possible, before or after a visit. Fear, lack of knowledge or just plain embarrassment may keep a person from presenting the true symptoms or complaints to the physician. In this case, everybody loses. Early treatment can be deferred if the diagnosis is delayed and the physician's time is not utilized effectively.

Mistakes, poor care, poor treatment and neglect can occur at different levels of the healthcare system. Another example: A physician on Long Island was found to be using one-time, disposable syringes on multiple patients which resulted in several cases of Hepatitis C among his patients. The physician was replacing the needle each time he used a multi-dose vial, allowing blood contaminants to be transferred from the syringe into the vial. Whether he was attempting to save money on syringes or genuinely did not believe that cross contamination could occur is unclear. When one of the patients filed a complaint with the Office of Professional Medical Conduct, the doctor was cleared of any wrongdoing but did agree to be monitored and inspected for three years. (26)

A Connecticut housewife and mother went in to a local hospital for removal of uterine fibroids. She died as a result of an artery being cut inadvertently in the operating room by a medical resident. The medical resident had a documented history of substandard work in surgery, supposedly unknown to the attending physician who supervised the surgery. In the recovery room, the woman was cold and pale and her blood pressure was dropping, all signs that she was bleeding internally. After a state investigation, the hospital agreed to pay a $15,000 fine and to hire a nurse consultant to review its procedures and recommend changes to prevent a reoccurrence. (27) The medical resident continued to practice at a different hospital.

A situation occurred in a Las Vegas Surgical Center when single-use equipment was re-used on thousands of patients. Over 40,000 people may have been exposed to Hepatitis B and C, as well as possible HIV contamination, when single-use, disposable syringes were reused and multi-dose vials were used at an endoscopy center. (28) In Nevada, the list of surgical centers accused of dangerous practices is growing. As of March 2008, four more Nevada clinics were being investigated for putting their patient's health at risk after a recent state inspection.

In New York, the Manhattan Eye, Ear and Throat Hospital was fined by state health officials after two women died from anesthesia problems for cosmetic surgery. The hospital paid a $20,000 fine and hired a consultant to evaluate the anesthesia department procedures and monitoring practices. (29)

Mistakes are also made at the medication level. It is estimated by the National Academies that approximately 1.5 million people are injured by medication annually and as many as 7,000 people a year die in the United States due to medication errors. (30) Whether in a hospital or home setting, everyone should be aware of what medication has been ordered, what they are taking it for and what it looks like. With more and more prescription medications being introduced to the market, the names are becoming increasingly similar. According to the U.S. Pharmacopeia, the rate of drug name mix-ups has more than doubled since 2004. (31)

The issue of medication safety starts when a physician orders a new medication. Simply ask what you are taking it for and for how long. You can ask if there are any major complications or side effects from this medication that you might expect. Your pharmacist is an excellent resource person for any medication that you are taking. Each drug is packaged with a product insert at the pharmacy. Most pharmacists will discard this and you will never see it, but you can ask for a copy and it will be provided to you. Be forewarned, the Product Insert contains EVERY known side effect of a particular drug. Most people will never experience any, so the faint of heart may not want to read the detailed information and may be better off just asking the physician or pharmacist for the major adverse reactions that are possible if you are concerned. On the other hand, I read about my mother's medications in depth each time a new prescription was written. I often cringed when she took a new medical prescription for the first few doses because she had so many adverse reactions in the past. I tried not to interfere with what was being prescribed but made sure a physician knew what her risk factors were. In a few instances, I called her hematologist (a blood specialist) to get his opinion on a new medication. When a hospitalist ordered one type of medication and she was already taking something similar, the hematologist informed me that she should not be on both at the same time. The hematologist was on his way to my mother's hospital room and said he would change the order. It was late in the day and I was heading home. However, when I came in the next morning, a nurse arrived with BOTH medications and quickly handed them to my mother. I stepped in and asked exactly what medications she was administering, only to be told BOTH. I quickly advised her that the order should have been changed by the hematologist the previous day and told her that my mother was refusing to take them BOTH until she called the hematologist and got this clarified. I also called the hematologist from my mother's hospital room. He advised me that he in fact did make the change the evening before. The order was never taken off the chart and had been missed. So a near mistake was averted. You have to remain even more vigilant in a hospital setting where several physicians may be ordering medications.

Take a notebook to the hospital so you can write down the names of the medications. Each time a nurse brings in a medication ask what the name of it is and what it is used for. Question any changes or omissions that occur.

Never take a medication in a hospital without knowing its name, dose and what it is for. If you don't understand, ask questions.

Every drug has the potential of causing an adverse reaction. Doctors cannot be expected to know everything there is about a drug. I always looked up all of my mother's medications and found many interactions with other medications that she was being given.

I once told a nurse on a hospital unit that my mother was not refusing to take a medication, but would wait until the physician came in to discuss it with her, the reason being the condition that it had been ordered for had resolved. Sure enough, the physician came in a short while later and my mother no longer needed that medication.

The week that I finished writing this book, I experienced another unfortunate incident with a physician's office. Several weeks prior, I went to a new female gynecologist for my annual pap smear. I chose her because she was "in network" and had been recommended several years ago. I brought along copies of my previous health records relating to my obstetrical and gynecological history. When the physician came into the exam room, she did not appear interested in my health history and did not ask me any detailed questions. I took my cue from her, but did mention my history of recurrent ovarian cysts with pain. She quickly muttered that my right ovary felt enlarged and ordered an in-office ultrasound for the next day. I was told that I would get a phone call from the doctor within a day or two regarding the ultrasound report and another call reporting the pap results when they were ready. Three weeks went by and I did not receive a phone call. I did, however, get a statement from my health insurance carrier stating that they would not pay $566.00 for laboratory fees on the date that I had visited the gynecologist. I called my insurance carrier and was informed the specimens (totaling four in all) had been sent to an out-of-network laboratory. I called the physician's office billing representative who stated they are unable to keep track which patients participate with which laboratories but admitted that their office uses three different labs. I know for a fact that organized, reputable doctor offices have lists of laboratories and which medical insurance carriers are participating with each. Occasionally, an office worker will misread the list and send the specimen to an out-of-network laboratory. I got nowhere with the office billing person, only more frustrated. I asked for copies of my laboratory results to be faxed to me, and even suggested that she fax me a medical release form so I could sign it and fax it back. The billing person stated, "We don't do that, I'll have the doctor call you." I guess she must have told the doctor an earful, as the next day the physician called. I barely opened my mouth when the physician stated, "Was that an edge in your voice?" I have to admit, I do get frustrated when I am billed $566.00 for something that I shouldn't have to pay for, but I was talking in my normal tone. Then I began to say, "Well, your staff......." The doctor interrupted me, "MY STAFF DIDN'T DO ANYTHING!" I was going to say, "Your staff sent my laboratory specimens to a non-participating lab and now I am being billed for it." The doctor then called to her billing person close by and I heard the billing woman through the phone, tell the physician that she called the lab "yesterday" and "took care of it." I then asked my pap and ultrasound results. After providing me with that information, the physician promptly and curtly said, "Thank you," and hung up the phone. Two hours later, I called the billing person in the same physician's office and asked for the name and the phone number of the laboratory where my specimens were sent. I like to follow up when I am legally responsible for the bill. With the phone number in hand, I called the laboratory. They stated there was no record of the physician's office calling "yesterday" or any day, and the $566.00 was still an outstanding bill. They further stated that the physician's office is the only one who can rectify this bill. I can only speculate that the office billing woman did not want to appear lax to her employer, so she lied about "handling" the bill and made me sound like the ogre. This issue is yet to be resolved and one more example of a lack of sensitivity, honesty and compassion in healthcare today.

Chapter 10

MALPRACTICE REFORM

"This research shows that the problem with medical malpractice litigation is not that too many undeserving people get paid, but rather that not enough deserving people get paid." - Tom Baker

We know that mistakes can happen and will happen despite the best efforts of all involved. The question becomes how do we compensate a family or person whose life is suddenly changed by an error in treatment or judgment. The current system seems to add to the business and monetary gain of the lawyers and does little to ensure that the same mistakes are not repeated.

A lawyer once told me that all medical mistakes are not grounds for a lawsuit. Medicine is not an exact science. It is taking the information that is presented, either verbally or acquired by examination or testing and attempting to diagnose it. Illnesses may need to be ruled out when the symptoms don't fit specific criteria.

Putting caps on medical malpractice suits has been written about in the past decade. Today, fewer than 2 percent of patients or families of patients who are negligently injured ever file a malpractice suit and even fewer receive compensation. Of those, only one in three involves no medical errors. Malpractice victims actually get only about 46 cents on every dollar awarded. (32) A survey of more than 1,600 physicians revealed that although physicians know they should inform on incompetent colleagues, about 45 % of them don't. (33)

Having said that, mistakes do happen, unintentionally. Most physicians or surgeons attempt to provide the best care and make the correct diagnosis. In 2007, there were several stories on television and in the newspapers about a hospital in Rhode Island that performed brain surgery in three separate instances on the wrong side of the brain. The Rhode Island Hospital was fined $50,000 and reprimanded by the State Department of Health after the third incident. (34) Obviously, this was not done intentionally, but changes need to be made to ensure that it does not happen again.

In 2000, the U.S. Institute of Medicine reported that up to 98,000 people die every year because of medical errors in hospitals alone. (35) Medical errors are not the only cause of death in a hospital. Many patients succumb to a hospital-acquired complication such as an infection. Hospitals are one of the easiest places to pick up a potentially fatal infection. Make sure that everyone washes their hands before touching the patient. Don't be afraid to speak up. I have seen the best surgeons get forgetful with this simple practice once they are out of the operating room.

Reform is needed to reduce the number of medical mistakes. According to Pam Villarreal, a policy analyst for the National Center for Policy Analysis, reform to the Malpractice System might include:

- Advanced setting of monetary compensations in case of death or unexpected disability based on the state workers' compensation system.
- Allowing compensation to be reduced for high-risk patients and high-risk procedures.
- Make information such as mortality rates for surgeries – more available to the public.
- Make the patient more liable by basing qualifications for full compensation on the patient's compliance with medical directives recommended by their physician. For example, adherence to diet, medication or treatment plan. (36)

Health professionals are not perfect and may also contribute to the medical mistakes and complications that may arise. Nurses, physicians, surgeons and anesthesiologists may experience dependency problems with alcohol and/or drugs. Many states, including California, have treatment programs for these practitioners that allow them to keep working throughout their treatment. "Alcohol and drug abuse are among the leading reasons for disciplinary action against physicians by state licensing authorities in the United States." (37) Patients are not privileged to this information. Several decades ago, impaired physicians would have to give up their medical license if they were caught abusing drugs or alcohol. This policy was changed to enable those who wanted help to seek it confidentially and maintain their career. Issues that need to be reported to a state medical licensing board would include suspected drug or alcohol intoxication while on duty, inappropriate touch and abusive or inappropriate sexual language. These are most likely not grounds for a medical malpractice suit in themselves, but should be reported. As a consumer, there is not much you can do but to trust your instincts on this matter. If you suspect that your physician may be impaired, you should seek immediate help elsewhere and document your findings. Report your suspicions to a state medical licensing board. The Federation of State Medical Boards has a link to various states here: http://www.fsmb.org/. Click on the State Medical Board Directory.

Another area of medicine that may affect our future care is the nursing shortage. In the January/February 2007 issue of Health Affairs, Dr. David I. Auerbach and colleagues estimated that the U.S. shortage of registered nurses (RNs) would increase to 340,000 by the year 2020. The authors note the nursing shortage is expected to increase by three times the current rate over the next 13 years. (38) Not long after reading that article, I went to lunch with two nurses with whom I had worked with in the mid 1980's. Although they were both younger than me - late 40's and 50, - neither had worked in the field of nursing in years, citing difficulty working with a group of "unhappy women." Out of my group of six close friends in nursing, only one continues to work in a hospital setting to this day, 30 years after graduation. One left nursing within the first few years and three left in their early 40's. One has gone back to working in a hospital but not in direct patient care, instead choosing to develop computer programs for nursing staff.

Reasons cited for the shortage in Dr. Auerbach's study included an aging pool of nurses who expect to retire, low enrollment in nursing programs, a shortage of nursing school educators, increased need for nurses, job burnout and high staffing turnover to name a few. I can honestly say I loved my work as a Registered Nurse, but over time, I witnessed the hospital being run more and more like a big business. The hospital administration seemed more concerned about the budget and maintaining their accreditation with the Joint Commission (JACHO) and less with the actual care at the bedside. At that time, the Joint Commission came for announced yearly inspections. Everything was polished and shined the week prior to the inspection in anticipation of the visit. I often thought that we should all be doing what we do everyday - taking care of the patient at the bedside and not put on a show for JCAHO. In recent years, the Joint Commission makes unannounced visits. Now, they are more likely to see the actual day-to-day operation of the hospital. The Joint Commission issues Safety Goals, which are a wonderful idea. Goals are usually a positive thing, but having a goal and attaining it can be a challenge when you factor in the number of hospitalized patients every year and the number of people working within a hospital who can have an affect on the care. Somewhere among my years of working at the hospital, mission statements came into vogue. Of course, they are common everywhere I look now. I often thought of them as rather silly. I had my own personal goals and morals as to how I wanted to work as a nurse. I didn't think a written mission statement would make a real difference in bedside nursing care.

A prominent concern in many hospital units is "the budget, the budget, the budget." Many top hospital administrators in the Northeast get paid six-figure salaries. When I was working at the hospital, consultants were hired to "trim the fat" at the patient care-level. They came in, made the work place unbearable for many and left after the damage was done. The bottom line was less time at the patient bedside and less hands-on nursing. When I trained as a Registered Nurse in the 1970's, nursing was more "hands-on." The nurse provided all the care and assessment of her patient. Giving the bed bath provided time to talk and assess your patient from head to toe. Healthcare is now fragmented. A patient care technician (nurse's aide) may come in to check the vital signs. When I worked on a medical-surgical floor, the nurse's aide did some of the patient assessment also. I worked on a 40-bed unit, with one charge nurse, two medication nurses and two nurse's aides. Each nurse's aide was responsible for 20 patients and had the medication nurse to work with her for assessments and treatments. The charge nurse usually was at the nurse's station for the duration of the shift, picking up medical orders and making sure they were carried out; problem solving and making sure everything got done. It was hard work, usually with minimal down time, running up and down the halls for eight or nine hours. It was a great learning experience and many new graduate nurses are introduced to working as a nurse on a medical-surgical floor, but many can only keep up the pace for so long and many nurses "burn out." Luckily, nursing is a profession with many, many opportunities. After getting the basic skills, one can work in a school, doctor's office or one of the many specialties within the hospital.

"In March 2007, a comprehensive report initiated by the Agency for Healthcare Research and Quality, was released on nursing staffing and its affect on the quality of patient care. Through this analysis, the authors found that the shortage of registered nurses, in combination with an increased workload, poses a potential threat to the quality of care." (39)

On several occasions when my mother was hospitalized, the staff did no complete body assessment. Her necrotic leg tissue was not examined or recognized for 36 hours, although she complained of leg pain. On another occasion, I removed her sock to check her foot circulation, only to determine that she had another blood clot that was obstructing the blood flow. I noted that her foot was white and cold on examination. On both occasions, I, as a family member, had to notify the staff to call the doctor. I shudder to think of how many issues are missed early because hospitals are unwilling to provide adequate staffing to allow their nurses to completely assess their patients. It seems we use the guise that we want the patients to be self-sufficient and do as much as possible. I always knew my mother wanted to be independent and would be so when she got home from the hospital, but she needed supervision and assessment in the hospital that was not provided.

According to AACN's (American Association of Critical Care Nurses), report on 2006-2007, U.S. nursing schools turned away 42,866 qualified applicants from baccalaureate and graduate nursing programs in 2006 due to insufficient number of faculty, clinical sites, classroom space, clinical preceptors and budget constraints. Almost three quarters (71.0%) of the nursing schools responding to the 2006 survey pointed to faculty shortages as a reason for not accepting all qualified applicants into entry-level nursing programs. (40)

I read an article that stated nursing schools in Connecticut were attempting to compact the nursing programs so that nurses could graduate sooner with their degrees to help alleviate the shortage. I certainly hope they don't compromise their admissions and programs to attempt to achieve this goal. However, anyone who has ever dreamed of becoming a nurse and didn't feel they had the means to achieve their goal may be able to qualify for some of the grants and scholarships that are now available to help alleviate the nursing shortage. The need for nursing educators is expected to increase to meet the educational needs of new nurses in the future. New nurses may need more emphasis on home healthcare as our population ages and we see the shift from hospital-based care to home care.

The changes over the past 30 years appear to be focused more on controlling the cost of healthcare and less on the actual role and integrity of those providing it hands-on.

There is no question that the field of medicine continues to change. We have more advanced technology, treatments and medications, all to help our population live longer, healthier lives. Even local retail outlets are opening in-store health clinics. CVS pharmacies and Wal-Mart stores have begun seeing patients in their in-store clinics. Nurse practitioners and physician assistants, who can treat a variety of ailments from colds to earaches, staff most of these clinics that are frequently linked to a local hospital system. This, along with generic prescriptions at the same location, can help to ease our emergency room and physician office crowding. Perhaps this will cut down on some of the serious wait times for true emergencies in our crowded hospitals and emergency rooms. One might consider going to one of these health clinics for a sore throat, flu shot or upper respiratory infection. Persons with ongoing chronic or serious health problems should be advised to be seen by their regular healthcare provider whenever possible. As always, ask for a written copy of any treatment plan or testing and ask for copies to be sent or faxed to your regular healthcare provider when someone is treating you other than your regular attending physician.

Chapter 11

PATIENT ADVOCATE

"The ear of the leader must ring with the voices of the people." --
Woodrow Wilson

Let's face it; we'd all love to have a doctor for a son or daughter. Wouldn't it be wonderful to have them coordinate your care, interpret the medical lingo and run interference for you? Unfortunately, most of us aren't that lucky, but having knowledge and a good friend by your side can be invaluable.

During times of crisis and stress we only hear a fraction of what we are being told. Likewise, the medical community does not seem to be listening to us. Time after time, I was my mother's advocate during her hospitalizations. I put information in writing and handed it to doctors and nurses. I reiterated the information in person. So many times, I felt like I was talking to myself and no one cared or was listening. Hospitalized patients are "sicker" than in the past 30 years. As patients go home sooner, those that remain in the hospital are there because they need more specialized care. They need total assessment - physical, emotional, and spiritual - with communication being key.

I can honestly say that this lack of humanity is not only in our hospitals but also in our corporate business world today. (But again, a hospital is a corporate business). I find it most offensive in the healthcare setting because we are supposed to be caring for people. When I encounter rude customer service representatives working at my telephone company, electric company or cable company, I often chalk it up to the younger generation and their lack of maturity. Somehow, I still expect more in a hospital. Why work in an environment that centers on people if you don't like to deal with people?

Chances are that everyone at some time or another could use a patient advocate. Most hospitals also have their own on staff if you need someone to step in to assist you get your needs across. Just ask for a patient advocate to be sent to your hospital room.

Ombudsmen may be available in your area to help you with specific complaints or concerns. An ombudsman is someone who will investigate and address complaints. The National Long Term Care Ombudsman Resource Center has a Web site. They provide a list of contacts of ombudsman in your local area and state. Contact information is located in the Resources Information section in the back of this book.

Ask a friend or advocate to accompany you to all doctor appointments. Bring your advocate into the examination room if you are comfortable with this, as this is where most of the physician interaction will occur. It is not critical that this person be a medical professional, but simply a good listener. Have your friend or advocate bring a pad and pen, listen and ask questions that you may not necessarily understand or remember. Devise a list of questions prior to the appointment and write them down. Educate yourself about any impending tests or scheduled procedures as much as possible prior to the actual procedure date. You can seek further information after the appointment at your local library, from another physician or from an outside health professional. You may want to use a microcassette recorder to record your doctor visits. Ask your physician for his approval and explain your reason for doing so. (That you want to be able to better understand his instructions when you leave the office).

The VNA HealthCare in Connecticut has initiated a Senior Assistant Program. By calling the VNA 48 hours in advance of an appointment, an assistant will accompany you or a loved one to a medical care appointment. The rates vary per hour, from $21.00 to $25.00 depending on the distance of the trip. This service is also extended for lab work visits, optometrist, dental or physical therapy appointments.

Remember that everyone is different and although your neighbor may have had the same procedure, it is not reliable to compare your procedure with his or hers. Every person is an individual with specific needs and individual factors that can affect the care.

You need to communicate any relevant changes in your health in a clear, concise manner. Include such information as symptoms, when they began, how they affected your sleep, diet and activity as well as your normal routine.

Being a patient advocate may entail talking with the physician on the telephone. Make sure that the physician has written permission to discuss personal matters with a designated advocate. Once done, the next hurdle is actually getting the physician to come to the phone. There are many variables in an individual physician's schedule. When possible, ask your physician when the best time and day is for you to reach him. Some days he/she may be in the operating room and cannot be reached. Often, Monday mornings are busy due to people becoming ill over the weekend and waiting for Monday morning to contact their physician's office. So if it is not an urgent situation, you may want to wait until mid-week to call. The day prior to a holiday or right after a holiday may also be busier times for you physician. Of course, in an emergency situation, you can call the physician's office telephone number at any time and your call will be directed to an answering service who will take a

message or connect you to the on-call physician. He/she may direct
you to the local emergency room for treatment when necessary.

Chapter 12

MEDICARE/MEDIGAP

"There are risks and costs to a program of action. But they are far less than the long-range risks and costs of comfortable inaction." - John F. Kennedy

Most Americans over the age of 65 years are familiar with Medicare, and many use Medicare as their primary healthcare coverage. In 2007, Medicare provided healthcare coverage for an average of 43 million Americans. This number is expected to reach about 77 million by the year 2031. Medicare is an insurance program, run by the United States government to provide health insurance for those age 65 years and older and certain disabled individuals. It was established in 1965 under President Lyndon B. Johnson. The money for Medicare health insurance comes partially from payroll tax deductions. The 1965 Medicare program had two parts: Part A - hospital insurance, and Part B - medical insurance. To qualify for Medicare, a person must meet certain criteria. They must be either a lifelong U.S. citizen who has attained age 65, a U.S. resident for 5 years, a disabled person for at least 2 years duration who has either collected Social Security or Railroad Board Disability payments, or those with permanent kidney failure or Lou Gehrig's disease.

In January 2006, Medicare Part D was instituted and offered prescription drug coverage. Part D was designed and administered by private health insurance companies. Unlike the original Medicare (Part A and B) of 1965, Part D coverage is not standardized. Each plan chooses which drugs (or even classes of drugs) they wish to cover, at what level of coverage and choose not to cover some drugs at all. Choosing the correct plan is confusing at best.

The Medicare/Medicaid system was never intended to provide comprehensive health insurance coverage. The majority of those enrolled will find themselves paying for supplemental coverage to cover the difference. Insurance to cover the cost difference is referred to as Medigap. Anyone over the age of 65 qualifies for Medigap insurance, even if they have a pre-existing illness. However, you must have enrolled in Medicare Part B within six months and sometimes there is a six-month period where the pre-existing illness will be excluded from coverage. Be sure to check with each company that you are contemplating enrolling with. If you have pre-existing insurance coverage with an employer plan, it is illegal to have duplicate coverage. It is possible to switch, but be sure to compare your existing plan and the intended plan carefully. Be sure to check with your employer to determine the duration of your health insurance plan in the future if you are covered through your employer. Get all information in writing whenever possible.

In 1992, Medigap plans became standardized under the Centers for Medicare and Medicaid but were sold and administered by the private insurance companies.

Also in 1992, Medigap Plans A through J were offered.

Part A, the least expensive and most popular, provides the least coverage and covers hospital stays if certain criteria are met:

- The hospital stay must be at least three days, three nights, not counting the discharge date.
- The nursing home stay must be for something diagnosed during the hospital stay or related to the cause for hospitalization.
- The care by the nursing home must be skilled if the patient is not receiving rehabilitation but has some other ailment that requires skilled nursing supervision.

Plans B, C, and D are more expensive and provide adequate coverage for most senior citizens. Plans H, I and J are the most expensive and provide the most coverage for senior citizens, including prescriptions.

Still, you will have to shop around to get the best rates for each plan. Costs can vary if you use a local agent (who may add a commission to your fee, however, the agent may be available to help with filing claims.) Rates can also vary based on your age and what state you reside in. Not all companies who offer Medigap coverage offer all the available plans. Be sure to check with AARP, AFLAC and private health insurance companies to determine the best rate for you. Determine if your rates will increase with your age or if they will be adjusted for inflation, which would mean a higher yearly premium. If you plan to move to a different area of the country, do not assume that your rates will remain the same. Generally, they will change.

Many employers are scaling back their retiree health benefits that were once very generous. The new plans being offered do not come close to covering what the old ones offered.

Some states are now offering Medicare SELECT Plans. These plans are basically a Managed Care Medigap Plan. You will be required to be seen at specific hospitals, clinics and sometimes, specific physicians, much like an HMO.

Medicare and Medicaid will not cover dental, eye care and glasses, hearing aids or routine physicals.

The Medicare program has been accused of being poorly administered. High volume of payments are paid out and many unscrupulous companies have been found guilty of taking advantage of the high volume and lack of close scrutiny of claims. According to the National Association of Medicaid Fraud Control Unit, in June 2008, two large pharmaceutical companies, Glaxo-Smith Kline and Novartis were fined in Alabama for defrauding Medicare by using a drug-pricing scheme. A similar situation occurred with CVS in March 2008. CVS pharmacies were supplying Medicaid patients with a generic antacid but were billing Medicaid for the more expensive brand name of the drug.

Estimates of wasteful health spending in the United States are in the billions of dollars. Some waste can be attributed to fraud while others to overpayments. The U.S. government pays private health insurance companies about 15 billion dollars a year to offer the Medicare Advantage program at a cost of 12% more over the traditional Medicare program. Interestingly enough, those covered under Medicare A and Medicare D never get to inspect their bills or payments made through Medicare. This encourages the practice of billing fraud. The President is encouraging U.S. citizens to enroll in the Medicare Advantage program. To pay for this more expensive program, he proposes that we cut 10% from the reimbursement that a physician now receives for caring for Medicare patients. So it would seem reasonable to expect that some physicians may limit the number of Medicare covered patients they will see in their practice.

Americans need to wake up and take more responsibility for their healthcare and related costs. We need to look at ways to save on healthcare costs and become more proactive in prevention and healthy living. We need to consider health savings accounts that can save money for our employers and ourselves. The idea of letting banks add health insurance products to their services has been discussed and has the possibility of lowering cost and adding competition to the market. The government needs to consider opening health insurance sales across state lines and adding more private health insurance companies as opposed to governmental programs.

As consumers, we need to monitor charges made on our behalf for medical services rendered, regardless of who is paying the bill. Most consumers do not concern themselves with medical billing when someone else such as Medicare or a private health insurer is paying the bill. There have been many instances of Medicare being billed for services not rendered, health insurance companies getting overpaid by the consumer and keeping the excess money and hospitals and physician's offices overbilling for services. Irresponsible billing and payments are not only fraud, but ultimately, cost us, the taxpayers. I spoke to a childhood friend who told me how her mother's estate was billed for several surgeries that reportedly occurred after her date of death. They had been scheduled prior to her death, but never occurred. The billing department of the hospital billed them to Medicare and there was a balance due which is why the daughter received the statement that she refused to pay. I know that I received a Medicare statement for my mother for a medical procedure that also reportedly occurred after her death date. When I called the hospital billing department, they informed me that they had another patient with the same name in the hospital at the same time. I really didn't believe their explanation and notified Medicare in writing regarding the bill.

In several states, a Medicare bus travels to various towns and cities to offer free counseling services regarding reviews of your Medicare coverage, prescription drug coverage, food stamps, home energy assistance and supplemental security income. It may be worthwhile to take advantage of this service to review current coverage and programs available.

Chapter 13

MEDICARE PRESCRIPTION COVERAGE

"Drugs are not always necessary. Belief in recovery always is." -
Norman Cousins

Enrollment in the voluntary Part D of Medicare took on new
significance in 2006. Those who were eligible had to enroll by
March 31, 2005, for benefits to commence January 1, 2006. By
March of 2008, it is estimated that 65% of Americans over the age
of 65 have enrolled in one of the Medicare D programs.

My own mother had wonderful health insurance coverage
but no prescription coverage. At that time, she was not taking a lot
of prescription medication; however, one inhaler alone cost over
$100. Fortunately, she was able to afford it and each inhaler lasted
over three months. She had asked me to look into Medicare Part D
for prescription coverage for her.

I made phone call after phone call to Medicare and never did
get any solid answers. What I did find out was that this system was

new to everyone and it seemed that the folks answering the phones were giving answers off the cuff. After much time getting through the telephone prompts and waiting for a live person on the other end, it was determined that there were about 50 plans available for my mother in which to enroll. To limit the choices, a potential enrollee must provide the names and dosages of all medications to determine the monthly allotments. That more than halves the choices. It is not an easy feat, considering that the ultimate choice is up to you and you want to get it right the first time or you have to wait another year to correct your error during the open enrollment period. Calling the local pharmacies was of no help. I finally determined that I thought she would pay more in premiums than what she was currently paying for medications, but I will never be sure about this one. It was all terribly confusing for a college-educated, computer-literate person. I can only imagine what the elderly had to work with to make their decisions. This system was not designed with the consumer in mind in my opinion. Luckily, I personally don't have to make that choice yet.

I can only wonder how much time, effort and money were spent putting this complicated system into place. If you have not signed up for this coverage yet, start researching the different options early. Call different pharmacists and check with the various plans to see which one best suit your needs and budget.

It certainly didn't help knowing that there was a penalty for enrollment for each month that you had not enrolled after May 15th of 2006.

Chapter 14

SAVING MONEY ON PRESCRIPTIONS

"It is easy to get a thousand prescriptions but hard to get one single remedy." - Chinese Proverb

Prescription medications and the pharmaceutical companies are a big business involving billions of dollars.

In 2006, a sales increase of 8.3 % was seen, which resulted in sales of $274.9 billion. (41) And yet, for the first time in 46 years, the prescription drug market dropped to its lowest point in 2007. Some attribute the 2006 climb to Medicare D and the 2007 fall to a combination of factors which may include more prescriptions coming onto the market as lower cost generics and medications pulled off the market due to contamination concerns and side effect issues.

Generic prescriptions usually mean a lower cost. Some insurance companies will only allow generics unless the physician orders it as "brand name only" specified on the original prescription.

Generics are an acceptable option if your physician agrees with the generic form of a drug. There is no generic form of a newer drug on the market for several years and it may be necessary to take the more expensive brand name. However, you can always ask your physician if there is an "older" drug on the market that will accomplish the same effect as the new one he recommends. Your pharmacist may be able to recommend a similar drug that is a different brand name or sold over the counter. You should discuss what you have been taking and what has not worked. The ultimate decision regarding which medication you take should be left to your physician.

Ask your physician if he has professional samples. These are actual medications given to the physician by the pharmaceutical companies to encourage them to prescribe their medications. There is no cost to the patient when receiving professional samples. There will be no handwritten instructions or dosing information dispensed with these medications and you will need to rely on your physician's verbal instructions unless you ask for it in writing. Don't expect that you will be able to treat a long-term illness with professional samples. This is not the intention of the pharmaceutical companies. They want your physician to prescribe this medication and for you to purchase it for long-term use at the pharmacy. It can be useful, however, to get you started on a day or two of a new medication and to determine if you have an adverse reaction to it prior to purchasing it. I have noticed a new trend in physician offices. Physicians are posting notices in their offices that they cannot provide free professional samples in place of a written prescription. I have seen such notices in several patient exam rooms.

Always ask your pharmacist if he is aware of similar cost-saving alternatives to the same medication you have been prescribed. Of course, you need your physician to change any actual medication order, but your pharmacist and physician should be able to work together. This situation worked well for me when my mother was ordered an expensive medication that was new to the market. The medication had a basic medication with aspirin added. By ordering the original basic ingredient and adding separate aspirin daily, my mother was able to save over $100 on her prescription. This was done with her physician's knowledge and consent.

"Over the counter" medications at the local pharmacy may also be a viable option. Simply ask your physician and your pharmacist. Many medications that were once by prescription only are now available at the local pharmacy on the open shelf. The cost may be lower than that of a prescribed medication.

Check your insurance policy, if you have one, to determine the maximum number of pills you can get in one refill. My physician used to routinely order my prescriptions for one-month supply. My pharmacist was nice enough to inform me that my insurance company would cover a 90-day supply at one time. The savings added up quickly. A non-generic prescription for 30 days would cost me $6.00 per month. The same non-generic prescription for 90 days still cost me $6.00. So I saved myself the time and effort of returning to the pharmacy every 30 days at the same cost. Over the course of a year my savings amounted to $168.00 for one prescription.

Some insurance companies also offer savings on mail prescriptions. This works well for medications taken on a daily basis over a long term. The principle is the same as the three-month refill plan, however, you simply order your three-month supply (or whatever limit your insurance company mandates), and they direct mail your prescriptions to your home at a savings.

Another way to save costs on prescriptions is cutting your prescription pills in half. Be advised that not all pills and medications should be split in half, crushed or broken. Splitting pills can alter the dosage especially if they are "time-release" pills, which should never be opened or split. The important thing to remember is that you still need to take the required dose that was prescribed by your physician. If he agrees to order double the strength, the pills will last twice as long. Again, it is important to check with your physician and pharmacist if this is a viable option for you.

It always helps to shop around at your local pharmacies, mail order suppliers and warehouse clubs for prices on prescriptions.

Prices may vary widely from location to location. However, if you are intent on saving a few dollars, the time and effort can prove itself worthy in the end. If you prefer to use one pharmacy but find your prescription at another pharmacy at a lower cost, ask your pharmacist to match the price. Many pharmacists will negotiate if you bring written proof of a lower cost from a competitor.

A large pharmacy chain may be useful when frequent travel is involved. Your electronic prescription records can be accessed at different locations of the chain pharmacy. Some people prefer a small, local pharmacy for a more personal feel.

You should always count the number of pills in your prescription bottle when you get home from the pharmacy. Pills are often or typically hand counted and errors can and will happen. The pharmacist may get distracted when counting out your medication. This is also a great way to inspect your pills, and familiarize yourself with their appearance so that you will note any changes from month to month. Some pharmacies are now using a machine that counts the actual number of pills dispensed.

In the past few years, I heard of busloads of American senior citizens taking hired buses to Canada to get their prescriptions filled. According to the Vermont Department of Human Resources, a consumer can save approximately 75 % of the cost of a brand name prescription in Canada over the cost in the United States. Interestingly enough, the same generic medication in Canada can cost much more than the same generic medication in the United States. President George W. Bush and the Food and Drug Administration have all gone on record as opposing legislation to import drugs from Canada. "Pharmaceutical companies also argue that current prices are necessary to fund research. They cite that only 11% of drug candidates that enter expensive clinical trials are successful and receive approval for sale. Proponents for legalizing the importation of drugs from Canada are primarily concerned with offering options to citizens, many who may not be able to afford necessary medication otherwise. They state that taxpayers already support research directly through the National Institute of Health. They also state that government currently grants pharmaceutical companies a federal tax reduction of 39% for this exact purpose. As a result, high prices are not only unnecessary, but are directly harming elderly, sick citizens that are usually on a limited budget." (42) Some drug companies have even attempted to make it illegal to allow Americans to purchase their drugs in Canada or even Mexico. There is no question that money can be saved when purchasing from these sources, but as of now, it is illegal to purchase any medications that were manufactured in the United States and were sold to an "outside" company with the intent of bringing it back into the United States. Currently, the FDA is not enforcing this ruling if these drugs are purchased for "personal use only" and many U.S.

citizens continue to fill their prescriptions by using either the mail, Internet, or personally traveling to Canada.

As you read in earlier chapters, drug manufacturing by well-known, large American pharmaceutical companies is occurring outside American soil and not without their own manufacturing problems. As recent as February, 2008, a New York Times story reported that Baxter International was being investigated for a link between a Chinese factory that was manufacturing a blood thinner that was possibly being linked to several deaths and allergic reactions. This medication is for use on the United States market. "Because the plant, Changzhou SPL, has no drug certification, China's drug agency did not inspect it. The United States Food and Drug Administration said this week that it had not inspected the plant either — a violation of its own policy — before allowing the company to become a major supplier of the blood thinner, heparin, to Baxter International in the United States." (43)

Counterfeit drugs are becoming more popular in foreign countries. You should exercise caution when purchasing your prescriptions. I have personally received numerous spam e-mails over the years offering prescription drugs for less - even without a prescription. I certainly don't recommend these routes, as you may never know what you are actually ingesting or in what amounts. Others simply attempt to mail order their prescription drugs from outside of the United States. Any prescription medication should be preceded by a written prescription after a visit with your physician. There are online pharmacies available on the Internet. Reputable ones require a written prescription from your physician in order to fill a prescription. If they do not require a written prescription, you should not use them. The National Association of Boards of Pharmacy has a Web site to assist consumers when purchasing medication over the Internet. They cautiously state, "Consumers should look for participation in this type of certification program (VIPPS - Verified Internet Pharmacy Practice Sites), as one method to help minimize getting bad quality drugs from disreputable sources." (44) Before purchasing your prescription online, it is advisable to see if the company has a phone number that you are able to call and speak with a live person.

In the U.S., a new drug or treatment must be tested and approved by the Food and Drug Administration. In the U.S. testing is done by giving a new drug to a limited number of people with the illness or condition that the investigational medication is intended to correct. Blind studies are conducted whereas one group is given the investigational medication and another group is given a placebo. Both groups are examined and report any effects related to the medication they are taking. These studies are usually conducted at large university teaching hospitals. When taking an investigational drug, your physical exams and related treatment are usually free, as well as the medication. Oftentimes you are reimbursed for your

144

travel for your participation in the clinical study. The medication you take most likely has not been proven to heal the condition for which you are suffering from, but it may provide a solution for those looking for help. Just because you volunteer for a study does not mean that you will automatically be chosen to participate. You must meet certain specific criteria to be eligible for the program. Check with your physician to see if he can determine where an investigational study is being performed and if you meet the requirements for admission into the program. This type of program usually involves frequent physician visits (usually with the physician helping to run the study) along with frequent blood tests and possibly other medical testing. Some of the well-known organizations that sponsor clinical trials or provide information include: National Institute for Health, Center for Information and Study on Clinical Research Participation, Centerwatch, Centers for Disease Control. See contact information in the Resources Information section in the back of this book.

If you are in a hospital, a nursing home or assisted living center, it is illegal for a nurse to administer any drug that has been brought into this country from another country. For example, if your family member purchased their medication from Canada, a nurse in the United States cannot actually administer the medication as it is considered to be imported illegally.

Anyone in dire need of medication in the United States should not go without. Don't be afraid to exhaust all avenues. Pharmaceutical companies have been known to provide medication for free in individual cases when no payment can be made. You can attempt to contact the pharmaceutical company directly or ask your physician to help you with your case. Your pharmacist maintains a list of phone numbers of pharmaceutical companies and may be able to assist you.

Others may get assistance through Patient Assistance Programs (PAPS). One such program on the Internet was located at www.needymeds.com. PAPs provide free or low-cost medicine to low-income people who are uninsured or underinsured. (45) On the Needy Meds Web site, some states, such as Maine, had a list of 24 resources available statewide for drug assistance, whereas my own state of Connecticut only had one, which was in New London County. This is only a small sample of what is available and those in need should investigate other sources through their physician, pharmacy and pharmaceutical companies.

Another resource on the Internet is RX Assist, located at www.rxassist.com. (46) This is a comprehensive site run as a Patient Assistance Program Center to educate those who need assistance with prescription coverage.

Another resource available for assistance with pharmaceutical costs is Together RX Access. They maintain an informational Web site at: www.togetherrxaccess.com.

Some of the brand name pharmaceutical companies will put rebates or coupons on their Web sites. Simply bookmark the Web sites of the manufacturers of the medications you take on a frequent basis and check back often for any buyer incentives to save yourself a few dollars. Some will periodically send you coupons in the mail if you register on their Web site.

Many pharmacies offer their own discount savings cards for prescriptions that you purchase directly from them. Some of these programs will charge you a monthly or yearly fee. The key here is to read all the information carefully to determine how much money will be saved. Once purchased, you may be locked into the program for a year. Not all pharmacy discount programs are the same, so it pays to shop around while bringing your routine medication list with you. Some programs may be based on financial income or other factors.

Many pharmaceutical companies, including Johnson & Johnson, Pfizer, Astra Zeneca, Eli Lilly and Janssen, offer discount cards. You can ask your pharmacist for assistance to identify which company to contact for specific drugs. Your pharmacist also has a reference book with contact information and phone numbers of various pharmaceutical companies.

Many patients feel that they have not been "treated" unless they walk away with a prescription in their hand. However, not everyone feels this way. If you are opposed to medication and would prefer to try alternative treatments, make diet or lifestyle changes, be sure to discuss this with your doctor. Perhaps the two of you can work out a time frame that is acceptable to see if any alternative treatment is beneficial prior to starting prescription medication.

Chapter 15

MANAGED CARE

"Cystoscopies, gastroscopies, biopsies. They can do three or four of those and make five or six hundred dollars in a single day but we get nothing when we use our time to understand the lives of our patients." - Dr. David Jones

The insurance industry is a big, powerful business. According to Medline Plus, a service of the U.S. National Library of Medicine, "managed care" are health insurance plans that contract with health care providers and medical facilities to provide care for members at reduced costs. The growth of managed care in the U.S. was spurred by the enactment of the Health Maintenance Organization Act of 1973. While managed care techniques were pioneered by health maintenance organizations, they are now used by a variety of private health benefit programs. Managed care is now nearly ubiquitous in the U.S., but has attracted controversy because it has largely failed in the overall goal of controlling medical costs. Proponents and critics are also sharply divided on managed care's overall impact on the quality of U.S. health care delivery. (47) The approval of this act resulted in the rapid growth of HMOs across the county. It changed the not-for-profit companies into for-profit. To someone working in the hospital setting, it appeared that managed care was the insurance companies' attempt at taking over the medical decisions once reserved for physicians. Not all HMOs are created equal. There are usually several tiers of health care coverage. Usually, the higher the co-pay or premium, the more coverage is associated with the policy. Just like Medicare Part D, most companies and plans have a once-a-year open enrollment when you can switch your plan. It is usually a good idea to pay for the best that you can afford, but be sure to read all the fine print in a contract before signing.

Along with managed care in the 1970's, DRGs came into vogue in the 1980's. DRGs are Diagnosis Related Groups. This was a system developed by Medicare to categorize patients with similar diagnoses and standardize how much hospital resources would be needed. Initially, a patient who was hospitalized was given a specific diagnosis classification. Medicare would pay a preset dollar amount to the hospital for that specific diagnosis classification. If the patient went home sooner, the hospital saw more profit; if the patient stayed longer, the hospital saw less profit. Since its incorporation in 1983, DRGs have been revised and expanded to several categories of DRGs to better fit today's complex healthcare systems.

With shorter hospital stays, the need for increased follow-up home care evolved. Someone at the hospital needed to be responsible to determine what the patient's medical needs would be after they were discharged from the hospital. And so, the role of the Hospital Discharge Planner evolved. This role really expanded in the 1990's. Increased hospitalizations with high-cost technological testing and treatments added to the cost of hospital care during this period. As a result, health insurance carriers began to restrict, deny or limit services, many times by including the phrase "usual and customary charges." It appeared that the insurance companies were denying or limiting coverage using this blanket phrase. They stated that they set usual and customary charges for each medical service at that time and if your physician or hospital charged over that amount, they would not pay. I remember this being a frustrating time with many phone calls to my healthcare insurance company. There was a feeling of helplessness as I could not control the fees charged by my physician or hospital nor could I control the amount covered by my insurance carrier.

As time evolved, healthcare organizations were forced to institute discharge planning into their organizations. Individuals were hired to interact with patients during their hospital stay, assess their health and activities and anticipate and coordinate the needs for discharge.   Many discharge planners are also responsible for communicating with insurance companies on a daily basis while a patient is hospitalized.   An insurance company cannot dictate when a hospitalized patient is to be discharged; that is the physician's responsibility.   Sometimes the physician and the insurance company do not agree and the patient remains in the hospital. Fortunately, we still receive the care we need, but the hospital often has to file and write appeal letters to justify the necessity of the hospitalization. Hospitals still incur the costs and patients can be billed for services.

Although this system seems to be working well on some levels, I have seen the wheels turn slowly for the patient who is sent home with complex medical needs. A patient may be sent home on Friday and discharge planners have set the wheels in motion for home health aides and visiting nurses services.   On many oc-casions, I have heard stories of home health aides simply not showing up or calling when they were scheduled. Usually a visiting nurse will come out to the home within 24 hours to assess the patient's needs after they receive a referral from a hospital discharge planner. However, it can take more time to get the system running smoothly, especially if there are complex problems or the hospital discharge occurs over the weekend. A dear friend of mine was on a blood thinning medication prior to surgery. During her hospitali-zation, her medication dosages were changed frequently and monitored by the hospital laboratory.   She was discharged on a

Thursday afternoon and no one had ordered a blood level to be drawn. So as soon as she arrived home, she had to contact her doctor to get a requisition for blood work to be drawn. Friday morning her daughter arrived to drive her to get it drawn. The results would be back late Friday night, and of course, her doctor would not be in his office. As she was not treated by her own family physician during her hospitalization, he was unaware of the changes in her medication. I could see she was concerned and frustrated. She decided to take the dosage that she had been on prior to her surgery, as there was no one to advise her. Fortunately, she suffered no ill effects while trying to determine which dosage to take. The Visiting Nurse arrived at her home the day after discharge but it was not until the following week that physical therapy was set up.

Although the Visiting Nurses can bridge the gap between the hospital and home they are only in the home a short part of the day. The nurse assesses and provides hands-on care and teaching for any related medical or surgical needs. This can include surgical dressing changes or specialized treatments. Most can expect a 30-minute to 1-hour visit several times a week. The home health aide can also be utilized. However, the amount of time is limited and restricted by Medicare or the primary health insurance carrier. Do not expect the VNA to provide around the clock companionship or care. Someone in the family needs to be involved in the care of a patient who has been discharged with complex medical needs. Family members are often expected to learn how to administer medications, treatments and perform surgical dressing changes in the home environment.

Sometimes patients are simply discharged too early or complications arise soon after the discharge home. This can result in an additional hospitalization if proper monitoring and treatment does not occur in the home.

Private medical insurance companies are also looking at new ways to manage healthcare outside of the hospital setting. In late 2006, I received a phone call on my personal cell phone from a company in Colorado. I live in Connecticut. The woman on the phone wanted to know if I wanted help from a registered nurse to manage my disease. I was astounded by this telephone call. I immediately got the name of her company and a callback phone number. Upon further investigation, I determined that my private healthcare insurance provider had contacted this company. With all the hoopla about HIPAA and patient privacy, I was shocked that my insurance provider could release such personal information to another party. Obviously, I denied any illness and declined their offer. I can only speculate that they were trying to manage my care to save my insurance provider some money. I contacted my insurance company by telephone and in writing to advise them that I did not want my personal information released to another party without my express written consent.

Personally, I have seen a lot of cost reduction and not a lot of improvement in the quality of care. Shortened hospital stays mean a vast savings to the health insurers. However, what happens when the patient with no medical background is discharged home with little or no knowledge of proper care and is expected to assess themselves? The Visiting Nurse Association has seen a dramatic increase in home visits in recent years. The VNA has been in existence since 1888. With decreased length of hospital stays, patients are going home with catheters, central lines and other medical equipment needing specialized care. The VNA is not going to be at your house 24 hours a day, so a family member or friend is usually expected to learn how to care for the patient. Mind you, most friends or family members are lay people with no medical training. If I was scared about the lack of proper hand washing and aseptic technique in the hospital, I am terrified of what goes on in the home behind closed doors. This puts people at greater risk for infection and other complications. What the VNA will do is come to your home, assess your vital signs, see if you need other resources and evaluate and treat your immediate problem.

My first interaction with the VNA was the mid-1990s. My father was completely disabled with Parkinson's disease and being cared for at home by family. The VNA sent a nurse's aide for 2 hours a day. My father needed to be spoon fed, but the nurse's aide was not allowed to feed him, because he "might choke," according to the registered nurse who managed the case. The nurse's aide could only clean the room my father was in and their schedule was unreliable. Many days, the aide just did not show up, without any phone call or explanation. Basically, the aide would sit and watch T.V. with my father for two hours while my mother ran to buy groceries. The time of their visits also varied greatly so they could not be relied upon to get my father washed and dressed in the morning. Many times, they did not arrive until mid-afternoon.

Years later, my mother had extensive leg skin grafts that needed bandage changes twice a day. I was with her every day at the hospital and at the rehabilitation center changing the extensive leg bandages with the nurses on staff. The plastic surgeon felt this was important as the staff rotated so often and I was the one consistent person viewing the skin grafts daily and knew the complex procedure. I would be able to assess the healing and intervene quickly if there were any signs of infection. After my mother was discharged, the VNA came to her home to evaluate her leg and her needs. I instructed them on the leg dressing changes the first day. The second day, a different nurse arrived and I gladly showed her the procedure. I expected a respite with the VNA there, after 12 weeks of doing the dressings and I was informed, "no, we don't do that, the family does." So I continued to change the leg dressings, despite my own complete physical and emotional exhaustion. On another day, the VNA arrived an hour after they had previously stated they would arrive and I had already changed the bandages. The nurse wanted to view my mother's leg. Of course, we refused as it had already been changed and I didn't want it disturbed again, which could interrupt the healing process. The only reason I allowed the VNA to stay was because they could order all the leg dressings and bandages and they would be paid for through Medicare, otherwise my mother would have had to pay for these expensive supplies herself. With both parents, I felt that the VNA was not providing the care that I expected and it was easier to do it myself. I am sure there are many isolated senior citizens who benefit from their services and many physicians who feel that their patients are getting close medical supervision when they are discharged from the hospital.

Obtaining nurse's aides through an agency or the Visiting Nurse Association can be a viable option for home healthcare. I do feel it necessary to advise one to use caution. As with having any stranger in your home, do not leave money or valuables lying around. There are caring, trustworthy and compassionate nurse's aides and there are some who are not so. I have heard from two friends that nurse's aides cooked food that had been prepared and left for the patient and consumed it themselves when they thought the patient was sleeping. I have heard of stories in nursing homes where patients were threatened by nurse's aides. Hopefully, these stories are few and far between, but it pays to be vigilant. Make sure that someone close to the patient is checking in often to be sure that everything is going well.

The VNA does provide numerous valuable services. They offer blood pressure, diabetic, cholesterol and general screenings as well as flu clinics among many other community and home health-based activities. They serve to educate and provide screening, which is so vital to early intervention to prevent future illness and disease complications.

Most states require nursing facilities to report all allegations of abuse or neglect to a local Department of Health. Some states even have online registries. It is best to check with your local State Department of Health to see if a person has completed the training and passed the test to work as a nurse's aide. Report any suspected abuse or neglect to the agency that supervises the nurse's aide or home health aide. Unfortunately, I have heard too many stories, time and again, to know that nurse's aides are still using intimidation of the elderly in nursing home situations. Sometimes those affected feel that it is useless to complain to management, as some form of retaliation often is directed back to them when a complaint is made.

Most ill or elderly people would prefer to stay in their homes whenever possible as opposed to being in a short or long-term care facility. Most, however, underestimate the actual cost of services for such home care, according to the Center on Aging compiled by the University of Connecticut Health Center. (48). The majority of Medicare money is currently going to long-term care facilities to care for long-term residents. Beds are usually full in these facilities with long waiting lists to get in. As our population continues to benefit from better healthcare, we can expect to live longer and the availability of long-term care beds should become increasingly difficult to obtain. Medicare coverage for in-home care is limited at present, but this may be changing soon with the advent of "Money Follows the Person," a federally funded program that has received millions in grant money to allow those needing Medicaid assistance to receive care in the home. The program was the brainchild of Joseph Stango, a financial advisor from Southbury, Connecticut, who maintains that the elderly and ill could receive better, less expensive care, surrounded by family in their homes, with the support of medical caretakers.

We now have more comprehensive home monitors that can transmit vital medical information through telephone lines. Some of these include transmitting cardiac rhythms, blood glucose and blood pressure information to physicians' offices from home. This enables those to be monitored at home, yet transmit the information at a scheduled time or whenever a concern arises.

Some HMOs have a gatekeeper. This is a primary physician who determines if you need the services of another medical specialist. I have heard of stories where the gatekeeper refused to order a consultation with a specialist that had detrimental results. The concept of a gatekeeper was to cut down on unnecessary visits to specialists. Individuals who have direct access to specialists in POS (Point of Service) HMOs do not make more visits to specialists than individuals enrolled in gatekeeper HMOs according to an article published in the American Journal of Managed Care. (49)

In a 2004 poll by the Kaiser Family Foundation, a majority of those polled said they believed that managed care decreased the time doctors spend with patients, made it harder for people who are sick to see specialists and had failed to produce significant healthcare savings. These public perceptions have been fairly consistent in polling since 1997. (50)

Chapter 16

HOSPITALISTS

"We have to ask ourselves whether medicine is to remain a humanitarian and respected profession or a new but depersonalized science in the service of prolonging life rather than diminishing human suffering." - Elisabeth Kubler-Ross

Hospital medicine in the United States is the discipline concerned with the general medical care of hospitalized patients. Doctors, Physician Assistants or Nurse Practitioners whose primary professional focus is hospital medicine are called hospitalists; this type of medical practice has so far not extended beyond the U.S. Dr. Robert Wachter in a 1996 New England Journal of Medicine first used the term "hospitalist". (51)

My local hospital promotes this program as "increasing patient safety, minimizing medical errors and expanding communication with doctors and families" as "some of the ways a group of specialists is improving the hospitalization experience." (52)

What does this mean to you? When you are admitted to a hospital, it is likely that the primary physician caring for you will be a "hospitalist." He or she is an employee of the hospital and does not have an outside office practice. They will coordinate your medical care during your hospital stay and communicate with your own private physician. You will not, however, see your private physician during your hospital stay, unless he/she is a surgeon or specialist who also has an office within the hospital. Some hospitals are still in a transition period with the hospitalist program and may allow you the choice to be treated by the hospitalist or your own personal physician. I spoke with several physicians regarding this relatively new trend in medicine. One physician travels to two separate hospitals each morning to do rounds on his patients. He feels that he is ultimately responsible for "his" patients. Another, an internist in the same city, also continues to see his own hospitalized patients, citing, "This is why I went into medicine."

Some of the concerns are that the physician directing your care does not know you as a person or your heath history. It is of utmost importance that you are able to communicate to this physician your complaints and needs, as well as your complete medical history as accurately as possible. This is when a written health history and detailed list of medications and your personal physician's names can be invaluable. This will allow the hospitalist to communicate with your other physicians if he/she needs more information than you can provide.

Personally, I have found this system frustrating. My mother who had multiple systemic health issues was hospitalized several years ago. The hospitalist was not receptive to my "suggestions" to call in her cardiology or hematology physicians on consult even though they both had offices in the building. These specialists are not allowed to treat the patient without a formal, written consultation from the hospitalist. Of course, when the situation became critical, consultations were called in.

The good news is that there is a hospitalist onsite at the hospital at all times. You may, however, see a different hospitalist daily during your stay, depending on the physician's work schedule. However, these physicians will communicate with each other and you do not have to restate your entire life history to the new hospitalist every morning. Whereas your personal doctor would come to visit you perhaps one time a day in the past, a hospitalist is usually available 24 hours a day/7 days a week. This system does allow your personal physician more time in the office to see patients and handle the large volume of paperwork associated with medical care today.

You'll want to check with your personal physician if he/she will be directing your care if you are hospitalized and how they will communicate with the hospitalist if he/she will not be at your hospital bedside.

The hospitalists work for the hospital and may have more incentive for getting you out the door quickly - ready or not! Some hospitalists are being offered monetary incentives by the hospital and/or insurance companies to move the patients quickly through the hospitalization process. Various formulas are used by hospitals, with many paying a base pay to their hospitalists. Each hospitalist may receive additional money for each patient that they care for. The more patients that are going through the revolving doors of the hospital adds up to additional money for the hospital-based physician. If hospitals are going to send the patient home sooner, there needs to be more support and care for the patient at the receiving end when they go home. The personal care physician needs to be more involved in providing adequate, thorough continuing care if needed after discharge.

Once I was discharged from the hospital on a Friday afternoon of a holiday weekend. The problems that incurred were lack of follow-up care for issues that were unresolved during the hospital stay and lack of physicians to direct my care during the holiday weekend. Additional cardiac testing was necessary, which could have been performed in the hospital but was not. This resulted in a one-week delay while I had to make a follow-up appointment with my cardiologist on a Tuesday and then schedule the testing as an outpatient, which occurred three days later. It took six additional days for me to be seen by my internist in the office for other unresolved health issues that were identified in the hospital but not actively addressed. It took exactly 13 days for me to get an antibiotic for symptoms that appeared on day one of the hospital stay.

A close friend had a similar experience when she was discharged on a Friday afternoon while taking a blood thinner. No blood level was drawn for several days prior to discharge and her own physician had not been involved with her medical care for the previous three weeks since her surgery. The hospitalist was no longer providing her care and did not want to order the dose of the blood thinner, and the next day was a weekend. The visiting nurses were to be involved but could not come until the next day and the patient was left wondering what dosage she was supposed to take. Fortunately, this woman was also a retired nurse and very resourceful in resolving problems. She was able to talk to her personal physician's nurse and come up with a treatment plan for the weekend that was effective.

Chapter 17

PATIENT RIGHTS

"Our lives begin to end the day we become silent about things that matter." - Martin Luther King

Each hospital has its own Patient Bill of Rights. The U.S. Advisory Commission on Consumer Protection and Quality in the Health Care Industry adopted a National Patient Bill of Rights in 1998. A summary is provided below.

Your rights under this plan include:
- The right of information disclosure.
- You have the right to accurate and easily understood information regarding your illness or condition so that you can make an informed decision.
- You have a choice of health care providers and plans.
- You have the right to emergency services care if your life is in serious danger without concern for your ability to pay or prior insurance authorization.

The staffing of emergency rooms has become more difficult in recent years. "A nationwide survey by the American College of Emergency Physicians in 2005, the most recent available, found that of the 1,328 emergency department directors who responded, 73 percent said they had a problem with inadequate on-call coverage by specialists, including neurosurgeons, orthopedic surgeons and obstetricians/gynecologists. That was up 67 percent from 2004."(53) Many of these physicians cited concern over getting paid, concern over lawsuits and disruption of their personal and professional lives as factors for not being available for emergency room patients. Many patients get evaluated in an emergency room and then need to be admitted to the hospital. However, many times there is no hospital bed available and the patient needs to wait in an emergency room for a bed to open up on a hospital unit. This leads to crowding in the emergency room, sometimes poor care and adds to the lack of beds in the emergency room. The issue of not enough specialists is even more precarious. If you or a family member need a specialist, such as a neurosurgeon, and one cannot be located to come to your assistance, you may need to be transferred to a larger hospital which can waste valuable time that is necessary for your care. Check local hospitals in your area to determine what resources are available for specialty emergency cases before you are in a crisis.

- You have a right to make treatment decisions.

- You have the right to know your treatment options and have assistance from others to make those decisions if you are unable.

Although in practice, it doesn't appear that all physicians agree with this right. "In a survey published by the New England Journal of Medicine, 63 percent of doctors said it is acceptable to tell patients they have a moral objection to treatment, and 18 percent felt no obligation to refer patients elsewhere." (54) This refers to treatments that physicians may personally consider against their religious beliefs such as sterilization, prescribing the morning-after pill or other known treatments. In the same survey, 8% of physicians felt they had no obligation to present all options to their patients. (55)

- You have a right to be treated with respect and nondiscrimination.
- You have the right to confidentiality of health information. With this, you have a right to talk privately with health care providers and have your health information protected. You also have the right to read and copy your medical records and change any inaccurate or irrelevant information that is contained therein.
- You have the right to an objective review of any complaint against a doctor, hospital or any other health care representative. (56)

Just because we have this Bill of Rights does not automatically mean that you will get the best care when needed. However, I have added a few pointers below:

- Do you know that you do have a right to view your medical records? Some may make it difficult to obtain the records or charge exorbitant fees for copies. As I stated previously, ask your physician as soon as possible for a copy.

- You have a right to say no. Please use this with caution. A wrong decision can cost you or a loved one your life. You need to make informed decisions. In case of an emergency, you may not be able to wait for a second opinion. Sometimes, seconds count.

- You have a right to good medical care. Don't accept or tolerate poor care. Within a hospital, if issues do not get resolved, ask to see the nurse manager, nursing supervisor, patient care coordinator or hospital administrator. Your doctor has the final say regarding the actual care that you receive. In nursing home and rehabilitation facilities, ask for a meeting with a panel of their health team workers. This may include everyone from dietitians to nursing administration and social services. Be prepared when you face a panel of administrators. Bring a list with you with the issues to be addressed. Whenever possible, document examples of poor care with photos and suggest solutions to the problems.

My mother had severe COPD and asthma. The hospital insisted on using their own medications whenever she was admitted and insisted that they did not have the brand of inhalers that she used at home. Hospitals can, however, get them in most cases, or allow you to use your own brought in from home if you have them identified by the hospital pharmacist. My mother seemed to do best with her own inhalers and we experienced this same issue when she was transferred to the rehabilitation facility. My mother also was accustomed to waking early and using her inhalers early in the morning. The rehabilitation facility had their own ideas regarding this. They scheduled the inhalers at 9 a.m. and then took her immediately to physical therapy to walk. However, she wasn't able to concentrate on walking because she couldn't breathe effectively. They mistook her difficulty as a refusal to exert herself to walk. They had never met her previously but were judging her. They also placed her on rapid rescue inhalers and not her usual long-acting inhalers. I actually had to call an outside pharmacy from my mother's bedside to talk to a pharmacist to confirm my suspicions. Having done so, I had to plead my case to the nurse in charge and ask her to call the attending doctor. I finally had to call the doctor myself and had the medication changed. Never be afraid to step on toes when breathing or other urgent health care issues are in question. Having done so, I then addressed the staff regarding the time of administration of these breathing medications so my mother would be at her best to do her physical therapy. I asked several nurses and no changes were made until I called for a patient conference. I went prepared and the issues were easily resolved. When I explained the action of the inhalers and how breathing took priority over learning to walk, it was an easy fix. I am still astounded that it couldn't be resolved quicker with fewer people. The physician orders the medication and it is usually the nurse's discretion as to the scheduling of the doses, unless specifically ordered otherwise. The nurses on duty should have been able to simply change the time of the inhalers, but chose not to. Instead, the staff was calling my mother unmotivated. It was so obvious that they did not know this courageous woman who was driven to keep moving every chance she got. She lost a week of rehabilitation because they did not adjust her medication until after I called the patient conference.

Chapter 18

HIPAA - The Health Insurance Portability and Accountability Act
of 1996 Public Law 104-191

"Privacy is not something that I'm merely entitled to, it's an
absolute prerequisite." - Marlon Brando

On August 21, 1996, Congress passed the Health Insurance
Portability and Accountability Act of 1996. Under this act,
consumers were given rights to protect their medical information;
provide and/or continue health insurance coverage through group or
individual health insurance plans; to fight waste, fraud and abuse in
the health care and health insurance industry; promote medical
savings; improve long-term care services and coverage and simplify
health care administration.

Your HIPAA Rights - in simpler terms:
- You have the right to see and get a copy of your health
  records. In most cases, you should receive copies within 30

days; you may have to pay for the cost of copying and mailing. You may not have copies of your records when information in your file might endanger yourself or someone else.

- You have the right to ask that any incorrect or incomplete information be removed or changed in your health records. In most cases, your health records should be updated within 60 days of your request.

- You have the right to receive a notice that tells you how your health information may be used and shared. Decide if you want to give permission for your health information to be used or shared for certain purposes, such as for marketing.

- You have a right to get a report on when and why your health information was shared for certain purposes.

- You can get this report for free once a year. In most cases you should get the report within 60 days, but it can take an extra 30 days if you are given a reason.

- You have a right to ask to be contacted at different places or in a different way such as through your office or by mail.

- You have the right to ask that your information not be shared with certain people, groups or companies. However, your provider or health insurer does not have to agree to do what you ask.

- You have the right to file complaints if you believe your information was used or shared in a way that is not allowed by law or in a way that you were not allowed to exercise your rights. Complaints can be filed with your provider or health insurer or the U.S. Government (Office of Civil Rights of the U.S. Department of Health and Human Services). (57)

I knew I personally didn't care for the HIPAA section regarding personal information very soon after its introduction. It seems to me that we are basically signing a paper that gives more rights to everybody to see our personal information. Have you actually ever read what you are signing? When I have attempted to restrict or refuse signing, I have been told that if I do not sign, I could not be seen by the physician.

Each physician's office has his or her own HIPAA papers to be signed. Some are quite elaborate, giving permission for your personal information to be released to their partners, (without naming their partners, of course) and anyone else they deem necessary, for whatever reason, whenever. I really feel that the medical office staff and hospitals are getting HIPAA forms signed "en masse" and simply filing them away without regards to any restrictions or limitations. I have placed written restrictions on HIPAA forms at one medical office that I did not want to be called or a telephone message left for office appointment reminders. Time and time again, my written request was ignored and I was called and a message was left.

I read an article on HIPAA entitled, "Health Privacy: The Way We Live Now," by Robert Gellman , a Privacy and Information Policy Consultant. He states that for any hospitalized patient, the possibility exists for 1,000 to 10,000 (including third-pay parties) to view your personal information. Some of those people include physicians, secretaries, medical residents, nurses, ward clerks, orderlies, nurse's aides, nutritionist, physical therapists, pharmacists, pharmacy techs, billing clerk, administrators, staff lawyers, accountants, public health departments, federal and state agencies and even law enforcement agencies in some instances.

The HIPAA privacy rules does not apply to many institutions (e.g., researchers and law enforcement) that routinely obtain health records. The rules add some formality and new procedures and they give them some new rights. Only two of the new rights are significant. First, the right to notice allows patients to learn how little protection health records have today. Second, patients also have a right of access to their own health records. HIPAA offers some other rights, but all are significantly limited or have broad loopholes. (58)

I remember one day when I was walking down the hospital corridor and I saw my mother's physical therapist talking to two men in suits at the nursing station. I heard a reference that clearly was about my mother and waited until the physical therapist came into my mother's room. I asked her the identity of the two men that she had been conversing with in the hallway. She relayed that they were drug representatives with the company that manufactures Lovenox, an anticoagulant that my mother was not even taking. The physical therapist was telling them about the incident with my mother's leg, which I felt, was a violation of HIPAA. There was no need for these drug representatives to know the detailed information that I overheard her telling. I know this sort of thing happens all the time when unusual cases present in a hospital. I believe HIPAA will do little to change that.

Hospital employees like every one else, love good gossip. So when the unusual comes through their doors, you can bet that tongues will wag. In early 2008, pop star Britney Spears was hospitalized twice in a California hospital psychiatric unit. Thirteen hospital employees were fired when it was determined that they reviewed Ms. Spears' medical records inappropriately. Twelve others, including some doctors, were also disciplined for reviewing electronic records. (59) In the past, if a "paper" chart had been used, it could have been kept under lock and key so others would not have inappropriate access to such personal files. However, when hospital charts are electronic, the possibility of a devastating loss of personal, medical information is possible through mechanical failure, malicious intent, or breech of security.

I reviewed a four-page HIPAA policy from a local hospital outlining how my personal information could be used. The obvious ones included the use of my information for treatment, for payment, for health care operations, (such as management, personnel evaluation, education and training, and to monitor quality of care). Other releases of information included the hospital patient directory, clergy, family members and several vague uses such as emergency situations or "as required by law." The list rambles on and includes that they can use my information for fundraising, appointment reminders, treatment alternatives, business associates, public health officials, governmental authorities in the case of suspected abuse, health oversight activities necessary for investigations, inspections and licensure, judicial proceedings, law enforcement, research, coroners, funeral directors, military command authorities, worker's compensation and disaster organizations.

So you can see, in order to obtain health care, I basically signed over my rights to my private information to just about anyone the treating facility deems necessary. I have given up my personal privacy rights so I could be treated.

Another hospital facility that I use routinely also gave me a copy of their HIPAA Policy. Again, this policy rambles on to state, "I understand that I have the right to request that **** restrict how my protected health information is used and disclosed for treatment, payment and health care operations. I further understand that **** is not required to agree to my requested restrictions." (60) HUH? Does anyone else see a problem with this? Again, we are told to sign a paper that gives more rights away than we get. To ensure complete privacy for a delicate matter, one would have to pay up front, with cash, refuse the HIPAA and refuse to release the information to the insurance carrier. I would suspect that many medical offices would not treat you without proper identification. Many, in fact, are asking for photo identification at the time of the appointment. This has come as a preventative for someone trying to use your identity and your healthcare insurance coverage on themselves. Identity theft, of course, is completely illegal, but has been done by desperate people over the past several years and is a growing phenomenon in the United States. By using someone's name, personal information and health insurance information, people have even checked into the hospital for surgical procedures. The problem comes to light when the real person is left with ruined financial credit or outstanding medical bills that they never even incurred.

For this reason, you should protect your health insurance information at all times. I am all for showing a picture identification at the time of medical services, but I do not use my driver's license and I do not allow a copy of my driver's license to be photocopied.

There are alternative photo identifications that can be used, such as government issued or non-driver photo identification cards issued by the Department of Motor Vehicle. Some credit card companies will issue a credit card with your photo on it, which also adds to the security of the credit card if it is lost or stolen.

However, there is usually a HIPAA Compliance Officer or Privacy Official that you can contact to request restrictions. Good luck with that venture. I've tried and my blood pressure goes up several points just thinking about it.

Recently, I had a positive experience with a HIPAA Compliance Officer. I attempted to call my physician's office, which is located within a hospital. I first spoke to the hospital operator and then asked for my doctor's telephone extension. I was surprised to hear a recording that stated, "Your telephone call may be recorded for quality assurance." I was shocked. I truly believe that a telephone-recording device does not belong on a telephone line where I am asked personal information, such as, "Why do you need to see the doctor?" Who would be listening to these recordings, how would they be stored, or erased? I was so shocked at the recording that I hung up the phone and dialed the hospital operator again. This time I asked for the HIPAA Compliance Officer. I was given a name and a phone number and my phone call was transferred. The HIPAA compliance officer picked up the telephone and I told him of my concerns. Some of my suggestions included an "opt out" if someone did not want a call recorded. The Compliance Officer was not even aware of any recordings being made but agreed to check into it and call me back. A short while later, he returned my call. He stated that the message on the phone line had only been in place for a week. (I was aware of that because I had been using that phone number in excess of 15 years). He also stated that no actual recordings were being done at this time, but stated the recordings were going to be made to check quality assurance of the hospital telephone operators. (I personally doubt this, as the warning message is heard AFTER you have already spoken to the hospital telephone operator and have given her a telephone extension in which to forward your call.) The Information Technology people responsible for the message and eventual recording were "away" for several days but he would relay my concerns that recordings on a hospital line were inappropriate and against HIPAA in my opinion. I further reiterated the "opt out" option for those who do not want their calls recorded. I did call the same telephone number the next day, and in fact the recorded message was no longer on the line. Months later, I called this number on several occasions and there was no longer a message regarding recorded phone calls on the line.

I had another experience with HIPAA while checking in at a physician's waiting room. I arrived for an appointment on a particular afternoon and a man followed me in the door of the doctor's waiting room. I arrived at the front counter and gave my name and my doctor's name. The girl asked me to state my birthday, which I did. I sat down to wait and the man behind me approached the window. He was asked to sign some medical release forms. A discussion ensued regarding the signing of the papers. The man then stated to the receptionist, "You do realize that I am a HIPAA compliance officer." She stated, "Yes, I still need you to sign the papers." Then he turned to me and stated, "Your HIPAA rights were just violated." I told him I was aware of that and further, "My HIPAA rights are usually violated every time I go to a doctor's office." We had a nice discussion regarding how more rights are given up by signing HIPAA forms than are protected.

Chapter 19

HEALTHCARE AND TRAVEL

Illness Abroad and Medical Emergencies in the Air

"A man travels the world in search of what he needs and returns home to find it." - George Moore

No comprehensive book on medical care would be complete without mentioning medical care while traveling. Unfortunately, your medical care may be compromised when you are traveling and you may be required to pay large fees up front for "out-of-network" emergency medical care. If you have health insurance, you may be liable for higher co-pay costs for out-of-network care or have no medical insurance coverage at all in a foreign country.

If you have serious health issues or concerns, you may want to consider health travel insurance, trip cancellation insurance and familiarize yourself with resources to get back to the United States in the event of a catastrophic illness while you are off American soil.

A good policy would cover international air evacuation and an air ambulance in the event that you are seriously ill or injured while traveling.

The United States Department of State maintains an informative Web site regarding travel abroad. Some of the tips offered on their Web site regarding your healthcare include:

Register your travel plans with the State Department through a free online service at https://travelregistration.state.gov.

Make sure you have a signed, valid passport and a visa, if required, and fill in the emergency information page of your passport.

Leave copies of your itinerary, passport data page and visas with family or friends, so you can be contacted in case of an emergency.

Ask your medical insurance company if your policy applies overseas, and if it covers emergency expenses such as medical evacuation. If it does not, and most will not, consider supplemental insurance. Medicare, Medicaid and Social Security will not pay for medical costs or prescriptions outside of the United States. The names of some short-term travel insurance companies that provide policies can be found at the Bureau of Consular Affairs Web site. See the Resources Information section at the end of this book. Another Web site that lists a wide array of companies offering health insurance in foreign countries including MedJet Assist (an air evacuation service for medical emergencies) is Insuremytrip.com.

Seniors may also contact AARP (American Association of Retired Persons), for Medicare supplement plans to see if they can purchase a short-term travel insurance rider. It is important to bring your insurance card, AARP card, Medicare card, in addition to personal identification cards, when you travel.

To acquire information about traveling with disabilities or handicapped access on cruise ships, hotels or various foreign cities, Access-Able Travel Source maintains a Web site at www.access-able.com.

The International Association for Medical Assistance to Travelers (iamat.org) can recommend English-speaking doctors at your destination.

In case of an emergency, contact the Consular personnel at U.S. Embassies and Consulates abroad or in the U.S. The Consular personnel are available 24 hours a day, 7 days a week, to provide emergency assistance to U.S. citizens. Contact information for U.S. Embassies and Consulates appears on the Bureau of Consular Affairs Web site at http://travel.state.gov. The U.S Embassies can also recommend English-speaking physicians in a foreign country.

Also note that the Office of Overseas Citizen Services in the State Department's Bureau of Consular Affairs may be reached for assistance with emergencies at 1-888-407-4747, if calling from the U.S. or Canada, or 202-501-4444, if calling from overseas. (61) The U.S. Consulate can help find a local hospital in a foreign land, notify friends and family at home or get money sent to the foreign country to pay for medical care. The cost of getting an ill traveler back to the United States can cost in excess of $50,000 according to the U.S. Department of State.

If a traveler is going to a specific location, they should familiarize themselves with the area before they travel. Certain localities may present specific challenges or threats to travelers. Some of these can include altitude sickness, which can affect respiratory conditions, illnesses or infections in the area, pollution or even a lack of medical facilities. The World Health Organization maintains a current list of illnesses or health threats on their Web site at www.who.int. I have actually had my personal physician locate a name of a hospital and physician in another country to which I was expected to travel in case I needed emergency medical care.

The Joint Commission (JACHO), which accredits hospitals and medical facilities in the U.S., is also responsible for accrediting facilities outside our country. Check their Web site prior to traveling and locate a JACHO-accredited hospital in the region you intend to travel. Print the information and bring it with you.

If you take medication, it is important to bring enough with you for the entire trip and then some. A good rule is to bring at least an additional week's worth of medication. A letter from your personal physician with the nature of your illness and the name and dosages of your medications can be critical in an emergency. Leave all medications in their original containers and never pack them in checked luggage where they may become lost. It is also advisable to check with the embassy of a foreign country of travel to determine if a specific medication is considered to be illegal in their country prior to your trip. A list of foreign embassies can be found on the U.S. Department of State Web site.

If you do find yourself in a foreign country and have run out of your prescription, go to a local apothecary or druggist and bring your old prescription with you. Many drugs that are by prescription only in the U.S. are sold "over the counter" in foreign countries. The pharmacist may be able to help you in an emergency situation. You may not be able to bring it back into the United States with you, depending on the medication. So be sure to check before attempting to do so.

The Centers for Disease Control (CDC) in Atlanta, Georgia, maintains a Web site at http://www.cdc.gov/travel. They can advise you to possible health threats that are endemic to an area or even vaccinations that are required before traveling to specific areas. Many vaccines take several weeks before they develop immunity in your body. Be sure to schedule your physician's appointment well in advance of your trip. Other vaccines that you may require are based on the destination, your age, health status and previous immunizations.

The CDC Web site also provides general guidance on health precautions, such as safe food and water precautions and insect-bite protection. The CDC also maintains an international travelers' hotline at 1-877-FYI-TRIP (1-877-394-8747) or by fax, at 1-888-CDC-FAXX (1-888-232-3299). (62) See also the Resources Information located at the back of this book.

There are many U.S.-based companies that can provide air evacuation/transportation for the sick or injured. The costs can be exorbitant in an emergency situation. Some travel insurance policies may cover the cost of emergency air evacuation, so it is wise to check prior to purchasing.

Medical emergencies can also occur during an air flight on route to your destination. Fortunately, serious illness or death appears to be a rare occurrence during flight, but it does happen. If you are fortunate enough, you will be flying over the United States and not a foreign country when this occurs. If your symptoms appear serious enough, the captain of the airplane will decide if it is necessary to land the plane at the nearest airport so you can receive medical treatment.

Many years ago, I was traveling to Hawaii by air when the flight attendants were walking up and down the aisles asking if there was a physician on board. The plane was over the Pacific Ocean, halfway between California and Hawaii at the time. After several attempts at locating a physician, I volunteered that I was a registered nurse. I was immediately taken to first class where a patient was experiencing mid-sternal chest pain, nausea and was very diaphoretic (sweaty). Any or all of these symptoms can indicate a possible heart attack. She had no medical history of heart disease and no other illnesses. The airplane did have a medical kit on board, but as a registered nurse, I was not allowed access to it. A stethoscope and blood pressure cuff could have been useful. I was only able to ask her symptoms, visually assess her and check her pulse. There was no place to land the plane, as I might have suggested to the captain of the plane when he asked my opinion. Without medical equipment, I was unable to determine if she was having a heart attack, gallbladder attack or anything else in between. Fortunately, the woman survived the trip to Hawaii and was taken out by an ambulance crew that met us on the runway in Hawaii. I never did discover what became of her.

Fortunately, the airline industry has changed their medical protocols and equipment since my flight to Hawaii in the 1990s. A friend of mine has been an American Airline pilot for more than 20 years. He is currently flying the Boeing 777 on international routes and has told me the airlines are now equipped with AEDs, (automated external defibrillators) that can monitor a heart rate and rhythm and provide an electrical shock to restart a heart in the event of a sudden cardiac arrest. The flight attendants are all trained in the use of the AED. Airplanes on the international routes are able to utilize satellite communications to speak with an on-call physician for guidance and devise the best course of action for the patient. In addition to physicians, the medical kit (referred to as the "grab and go") onboard an aircraft can now be accessed by registered nurses and emergency medical technicians under the direction of the on-call physician. The flight manual instructs the captain of the airplane to ascertain key information prior to calling the physician. Some of these are:

Is the person alert, awake or unresponsive?

What is the age and gender of the person?

Is there any known medical history?

Is the person taking any medication?

What are the symptoms?

Is there a health care professional attending to the patient or on board the plane?

The in-flight manual also directs the captain to divert the airplane for landing if they are unable to contact the physician on-call, there is no physician on board and the person exhibits any of the following symptoms:

- prolonged unconsciousness;
- uncontrolled bleeding;
- persistent pain - especially chest pain;
- persistent loss of function of an arm, leg, face or speech (symptoms of a stroke);
- persistent difficulty breathing; and
- required use of the Auto External Defibrillator (AED).

After September 11th, 2001, pilots do not come out of the cockpit for any reason to interact with passengers, so the captain of the airliner will rely on information provided to him by the flight crew and information he receives from the on-call physician. The captain that I spoke with told me that in over 20 years, there was only one incident of chest pain on board when he was piloting and there was also a cardiologist on board the same flight who did not feel the need was imminent to land the plane.

International air routes have additional guidelines and restrictions for landing a plane in a medical emergency. Each airliner has a manual onboard with specific international airports that can be used in a medical emergency. It is up to the captain of the airplane to make the decision whether or not to "put the plane down." This decision is never taken lightly. Many factors must be taken into consideration. In the event of an unexpected landing in a foreign country, passengers and crew need to be housed and fed, all at a great expenditure. Once landed in a foreign country, a plane can be held on the ground for several days before being granted permission to leave. If the trip is an extended one, the flight crew may need to be replaced by a new crew that is flown in.

Airliners have the ability to take off with a heavier load than which they can land. In order to make an emergency landing, some thousands of pounds of jet fuel may need to be jettisoned off. This adds additional costs for the airline. Not all airports have adequate runways to land a jumbo jet, so airliners must be diverted to an airport that is suitable to the size of their aircraft. The proximity of a hospital to an airport must also be factored in. Passenger airplane manuals have a list of prior-authorized airports in which to divert in the case of a medical emergency. It appears that the airlines are taking in-flight illness seriously and are making every effort to keep their passengers alive until they can get them to expert medical care.

When traveling to foreign countries, you may want to consider bringing along the following items:

ace bandage

alcohol-based hand sanitizer

antacid

antibacterial ointment

antibiotic (broad spectrum) - ask your physician if a prescription is
      appropriate

antihistamine

band-aids

cortisone cream

current prescription medications (enough for the trip and an
      additional weeks worth)

decongestant

diarrhea medication

laxative

medication for minor aches/sprains/strains

thermometer

tweezers

In addition to the above, don't forget an additional pair of eyeglasses or hearing aid battery if you need these, as well as sunscreen and insect repellent.

If you have complicated health issues, it is even more important to bring copies of your medical records with you when you travel. I choose to carry a few "choice" medical records with me when I go out of town even for a few hours. I carry a folder with copies of my latest cardiac testing, such as stress test, echocardiogram and latest EKG, as well as blood test results. My folder also contains a detailed health history and medication history. On the front of my folder are the names of my physicians and their phone numbers.

In addition to packing your daily medications, it is advisable to include a list with both the brand name and the generic name of any medication that you take. You may also want to consider having your physician write out a prescription for you to take with you. If you rely on prescription narcotics or utilize a syringe on a regular basis, have your physician write a letter stating the medical necessity and carry it on you at all times.

Your list should also include your blood type if known, your known allergies to medication or other substances, a copy of your health insurance card, copy of your passport, a contact list of relatives that are not traveling with you.

If you have any medical devices implanted in you, such as pacemakers, metal hips or have been treated with radioactive isotopes, you should have your physician document this information in writing and bring this information with you. Medical procedures involving radioactive isotopes may set off radiation alarms at public transportation locations or at large public venues that use security screening devices. Documented examples of this occurred at a Manhattan, New York, subway stop. A man had been treated three weeks prior with radioactive iodine for a hyperactive thyroid. Similar cases have occurred weeks after patients stopped radiation therapy for cancer.

If you need supplemental oxygen to travel, most airlines will allow you to bring certain pre-approved oxygen concentrators on board the aircraft. Be sure to check with the airline well in advance to be sure that the unit you have is approved for use on their planes. You will not be permitted to bring or check-in any supplemental oxygen cylinders on any of the airlines.

Don't forget to use caution while consuming water or unwashed fruits and vegetables in foreign countries. In countries such as Mexico, you will want to avoid tap water and beverages with ice cubes. Ask for your beverage in its original, unopened bottle. Avoid uncooked or unpeeled food in developing countries.

Chapter 20

CRUISE SHIP TRAVEL

Seasickness

"All journeys have secret destinations of which the traveler is unaware." - Martin Buber

Many of us tuned in to the "Love Boat" on television when we were growing up and watched Doc Bricker in his calm, warm, affectionate manner handle any medical emergencies that came up.

Unfortunately, this is not always true to life. Many cases have made the news when American travelers on cruise ships became seriously ill or injured onboard. Many claimed that medical care was unpredictable, undiagnosed or lacking in other ways. Most people anticipating their relaxing vacation don't consider their health needs or health care available on a ship.

According to an expose by ABC News on their popular show, "20/20," "the doctor is part of the crew, but the cruise line claims no responsibility for the doctor's actions," said Miami

Attorney, Charles Lipcon (63). Lipcon goes on to state that in the event that the physician on board doesn't perform the proper care, the cruise ship will disavow all responsibility. Several cases were cited that passengers who were severely injured onboard by a fall were not properly diagnosed or cared for. This led to the death of one woman and delayed brain surgery for another.

Adding insult is the small print hidden on the cruise ship ticket that disavows responsibility of the cruise line in the event of such cases. Many cruise ships are registered to foreign ports such as Panama, Liberia or the Bahamas. (Just because they are based out of a United States port does not mean they are governed by U.S. rules and regulations). Their staff, including the medical staff, may also be foreigners and are independent contractors. These physicians and nurses may rotate through various cruises and attempting to locate them after an incident can be very difficult. One article said, "They get the same immunity from conviction when it comes to deaths onboard their ships as foreign embassy delegates have in New York City." (64)

In June 2006, a woman died on a cruise ship after most likely contracting the Norovirus. Her vomiting was so severe that she tore a hole in her esophagus. After more than eight visits to the ship's Ukrainian doctor, the woman died. At one of the ports of call, health inspectors had boarded the ship and this same doctor neglected to tell the health inspectors of the death onboard. (65)

In another case, a man complained of classic heart attack symptoms while on a three-week cruise. He had chest pain and pain in his left arm. The ship's doctor diagnosed him as having indigestion. A short time later, he had a heart attack and was revived by several passengers, who were practicing physicians in the U.S., using a defibrillator found onboard the ship. Fortunately, the man survived. He sued the cruise line for medical malpractice; however, it was thrown out of court. The court then ordered the man to pay the cruise line's attorney fees of $50,000, while refusing to provide contact information for the doctor who went back to his native land. (66) Cruise ships are not legally liable for the actions of the physicians on board nor does maritime law require cruise ships to provide medical care for the passengers.

In December 2007, a cruise ship off the coast of Mexico had a teenage passenger on board ship that experienced a ruptured appendix. A United States Navy ship about 500 miles away on a training session responded to a distress call by the cruise ship for assistance. An appendectomy was performed on the Navy ship, which had a surgical facility on board. Most cruise ships do not have surgeons or surgical facilities onboard.

In September 2007, a wrongful death lawsuit was filed on behalf of William Kerr, the spouse of the late Helen Kerr who died as a result of alleged wrongful treatment on a cruise ship. Allegedly, Mrs. Kerr had a large amount of fluid in her lungs. When she sought treatment at the cruise ship infirmary, she was given large amounts of additional fluids intravenously. This would not be an appropriate treatment and can cause respiratory failure similar to drowning. The case goes on to state that the captain of the ship would not allow for an air evacuation citing the itinerary and budget of the ship. (67)

This article does cite that in the past year, the number of passengers airlifted off cruise ships seems to have increased, occurring several times a month now. This is encouraging news to the thousands who travel on cruise ships yearly and experience a sudden or serious illness. Unfortunately, nothing can be done to ease the suffering of those who have already died but we need legislation and protection for cruise ship passengers who board looking for a fun filled or relaxing vacation.

If the nurses and physicians were mandated employees of the cruise lines, then the cruise lines would be held accountable for their actions or lack thereof. All relevant information pertaining to the physician, his country of licensure, contact information in his/her home country should be furnished to all passengers who come in contact with him/her during the duration of their cruise. I can only hope that these experiences will become less prevalent as the cruise ships that cater to millions of Americans, work to protect their image.

Even "slip and fall" injuries on a cruise ship can be costly to the passenger, including medical treatment and follow-up care by a personal physician. Cruise ships are not known for compensating for injuries sustained on a cruise.

Before booking your cruise, you can call ahead and ask the representative if their cruise line uses the accepted guidelines of the American College of Emergency Physicians. If they state that they do not, this may be a red flag to check other cruise lines. Even if they say yes, this is no guarantee that you would receive quality care if necessary.

If I felt I had a true medical emergency on a cruise ship and was not receiving proper care, I would either use the ship phone to call a U.S. Consulate or get off the ship at the next port and call a U.S. Consulate from there. It is better to be safe than sorry and to get the proper emergency care while there is still time.

Fortunately, a serious illness or injury on a cruise ship is a rare event, but it is projected that approximately 20 people die per year on cruise ships, mostly from heart attacks. (68)

Chapter 21

TIME FOR A NEW DOCTOR? A NEW HOSPITAL? A NEW
EMERGENCY DEPARTMENT?

"To me the ideal doctor would be a man endowed with profound
knowledge of life and of the soul, intuitively divining any suffering
or disorder of whatever kind, and restoring peace by his mere
presence." ~Henri Amiel

Factors to Consider

Not all personalities are a perfect fit, and we certainly don't
live in a perfect world. But unless there is some large personality
conflict, you may want to rethink changing your medical provider.

Our insurance carriers direct many people with health
insurance to specific physicians. We may only be allowed to see
participating doctors in our insurance plan for maximum insurance
coverage. Of course, you are always free to go out of network, but

be sure to check with your insurance carrier to see what balance you will be responsible for, prior to making an appointment.

Some physicians or surgeons may have outstanding diagnostic or surgical skills but just don't relate well with the small talk in the office. This can be a good working relationship as long as the physician/surgeon is willing to listen to the vital information he needs to get a diagnosis. It is important that the physician or surgeon takes a thorough medical history of not only yourself, but of your immediate family (mother, father, siblings and children). Write down this information before your appointment and bring it with you.

Many times, it is not the physician who has the communication problem. Patients may feel too embarrassed to honestly disclose their complaints, lifestyle or symptoms. Of course this can seriously affect your treatment. Without all the relevant information, the physician may not be able to make a proper diagnosis. Believe me, whatever you say will not shock your doctor. He has probably heard it all before and then some.

And yes, there are some physicians who are poor communicators. In this instance, you need to be honest and just tell him that you do not understand and need further explanation. I have heard of this complaint time and time again. I do think that physicians genuinely understand the importance of explaining their findings or treatment, and make an effort to use language that is easily understood by those who do not work in the medical field. You can ask the physician if he has an assistant, nurse or other medically trained person on staff to explain it to you in more detail. If you do not understand the importance of a certain medication, you might take it incorrectly or for a shorter period of time. I have also seen this first-hand. Elderly people will tell me that they stopped taking a specific medication because they didn't understand how long they should take it. Your pharmacist is an excellent resource person; so don't hesitate to talk to him/her when picking up your prescription. They can educate you about a specific medication, but cannot change anything the physician has written on the original prescription or advise you how long you need a specific medication unless it is written as such. However, if you find yourself in a situation where the physician doesn't seem to understand you and your needs and you cannot understand his instructions, it may be time to seek another physician.

I have to admit that I have met a few physicians who were extremely poor communicators, but fortunately, they are few and far between. If you recall, I discussed earlier the case of my relative who had to see a surgeon who proclaimed himself the "Whipple King." (The Whipple procedure is the surgical removal of the head of the pancreas, a portion of the bile duct, the gallbladder and the duodenum. Sometimes, a portion of the stomach is also removed.) My relative was not able to get past this surgeon's attitude and successfully had her surgery performed by a partner of the "Whipple King."

Some patients may feel slighted about the actual time spent with the doctor, especially after a prolonged wait in the waiting room. I personally have had this experience many times; however, when it was "my turn" with the physician, apologies were made for the lengthy wait and I was given the full attention of the physician. Some medical specialties and practices have their physicians covering emergency cases during the same hours they are scheduled to see patients in the office. That may necessitate the physician leaving the office for an extended period of time to attend to the emergency. Of course, those left in the waiting room will continue to wait. Other times, a more acutely ill patient will need to be squeezed into the daily schedule for a sudden illness or injury.

A friend of mine has been seeing the same physician for years. The problem is the wait time between the waiting room and getting into the examination room. This physician often leaves his patients waiting for hours at every scheduled appointment. My friend's solution was to schedule the appointment and have the office call her at home 15 minutes before she was to be seen. The physician's office staff was agreeable to this solution and she was fortunate enough to live close by. Obviously, this solution would not work well for everyone and not every physician's office would be agreeable to calling their patients at home 15 minutes prior to their appointments. And of course, what do you do with your time for hours while you are "on call" for your appointment? This solution works well for my friend and she knows this will occur at each appointment and accepts it.

Due to rising malpractice costs, many physicians have formed practice groups, which is much different from the single family doctor that many of us had as children. Coupled with this, many privately owned physician groups or hospital-based physician groups are mandating the number of patients that must be seen in one day. I asked several physicians and they were reluctant to acknowledge this, but did with the understanding that they would not be named. The decrease in medical insurance reimbursement is seen to play a key role in this. For example, some physicians may be required to see up to 30 patients a day during their office hours. During a ten-hour work- day, that would average out to about 20 minutes per patient. And of course, that is if there are no emergencies or complex problems or issues that arose. So you can see that you need to go into your appointment prepared. Mandating the number of patients seen appears to be a common trend that is growing. A favored physician of mine had worked at a large university teaching center for over 20 years. Upper administration repeatedly informed the physician specialists on staff that they had to see more patients. As a world- known specialist, my physician felt that she would be compromising the care of her patients by agreeing to these terms. She argued that her patients had complex and diverse medical problems and soon left to go to a smaller practice at another hospital.

I would also caution patients not to change physicians based on one negative encounter. Remember that there are many variables in health care. Perhaps there was poor communication regarding a problem or issue from the patient, the physician did not get a message correctly, the physician was having a bad day (hey, they are human, too) or the problem was complex and not easily diagnosed. However, if a continuing pattern arises, or a health issue is not taken seriously and the patient and physician are unable to communicate effectively, it may be time for a change of physicians. I heard of a woman who received extremely upsetting news from a well-known surgeon. In talking with her friends, she related that she did not like this surgeon at all. As time went on, the woman had major surgery for cancer by the very surgeon she had complained about. She later reported to her friends that she held the surgeon in high regard and felt her to be very compassionate as well as skilled. Perhaps the patient's first impression was a reaction to the devastating news delivered by the surgeon and not the surgeon herself.

In the beginning chapters of this book I explained the training that is required to become a physician or surgeon. I also mentioned that when looking for a physician it is helpful to check if the physician is board certified. This means the physician has taken and passed an exam given by a medical specialty board in a particular area or field of medicine. This implies that the physician has mastered the knowledge in his field and is considered a specialist.

The American College of Physicians maintains a Web site, which provides helpful information for consumers. Likewise, the American Board of Medical Specialties and the American College of Surgeons allows you to see which doctors are board-certified and which surgeons are members. A surgeon will have the letters, FACS, after his name if he/she is a member of the American College of Surgeons. See the Resources Information section at the end of the book for Web site information. If a physician is board eligible, it may mean that they did not take the required boards for certification or did not pass the exam.

Find out what medical school and residency program the physician attended. Preferably, you'd look for one that attended an accredited medical school and completed their residency at a qualified teaching hospital. This is not always the case. Be assured that if they are practicing medicine in the United States, they have passed proficiency exams to enable them to do so. With more and more foreign physicians practicing medicine today, we will continue to see more who were schooled outside of the United States.

Again, your choice may be limited based on your medical insurance coverage. You may need to see your primary care provider who acts as a gatekeeper before you are allowed to see a specialist. Usually, the gatekeeper physician in this case, will have the name of a specific specialist for you to see. However, this may not be set in stone either. You can ask why a particular specialist was chosen. Perhaps you have heard from friends or family of a different specialist. If that person is in your health insurance plan, you should be allowed to see that person.

Another factor to consider when choosing a physician is which hospital he or she is affiliated with. This is referred to as privileges. It is important that the hospital that your physician utilizes be JACHO accredited. This increases your chances that everything at the hospital is running as smoothly and safely as it possibly can. You should call the physician's office prior to your first appointment to determine which hospitals he or she has privileges at. If you are hospitalized as an inpatient, will the physician come to the hospital to direct your care? Does the physician let a hospitalist care for you as an inpatient? If most of your doctors participate with one hospital in particular, you may want to consider a doctor that also has privileges at the same facility. This can make it easier for the physicians to communicate or access your lab work. This does not bind you, however. I have many physicians around the state who practice at different hospitals. Most, if not all, provide me with copies of lab work, test results and even office notes so that I can bring them to subsequent appointments with the other physicians. I do this simply because these are the physicians who I trust, feel most comfortable with and can communicate with.

Some factors that you may want to consider when choosing a hospital:

- Is it participating with your health insurance provider?
- Is it accredited by the Joint Commission on Accreditation of Healthcare Organizations (JACHO)?
- Do they employ hospitalists or will your own physician treat you in the hospital?
- Do they treat the condition that you have at this facility? Smaller hospitals may not do cardiac catheterizations, for example.
- Does the institution appear neat and orderly? Talk to others who have visited or been admitted there.
- Is the hospital modernized? Modern hospitals are now using electronic charting and computers for physician orders as well as bar code scanners for identification.
- Is the hospital associated with a major medical university?
- Is it a teaching hospital that utilizes medical residents and fellows?

In addition to in-hospital care, facilities and services, it can be important to know if your physician has a preference which Emergency Department you visit and if he/she will treat you there. Many physicians will allow the Emergency Department physician to manage your care until you are sent home or admitted. Some important factors when choosing an Emergency Department can include:

- The distance from your injury or accident to the Emergency Department.
- Will your physician provide your health care or will he designate it to the Emergency Department physicians?
- Is the Emergency Department participating in your health plan? (In a life-threatening emergency, it is important to seek care regardless of cost or distance. Many insurers recognize this and will make allowances).
- Are the Emergency Department physicians board certified in Emergency Medicine?
- Is the Emergency Department accredited by JACHO?
- Are there specialists available on all days, at all hours? Some ERs do not have pediatric, plastic surgeon or other specialized physicians available on call. Are they willing to call in a specialist for a consultation?
- Are they trauma center rated?

- Are they staffed to do diagnostic testing on all days at all hours?

Several reliable Web sites are available for consumers to check hospital accreditation, ratings and services.

The first check is to confirm that the institution is accredited by JCAHO and is in good standing. This can be done on the Joint Commission-sponsored Web site: www.qualitycheck.org. Simply submit your zip code, the hospital zip code or name of the hospital you wish to check.

Other Web sites to check and compare hospitals for quality and safety issues are maintained by the U.S. Department of Health and Human Services at: www.hospitalcompare.hhs.gov and the Leap Frog Group at: www.leapfroggroup.org.

Physicians all practice in their field in their own individual style. Some elderly patients relate better to a physician who simply tells them what they need to do. These patients may have grown up in the era of when the physician was a paternalistic figure who told them what to do and they did not need or want to know more or question it. On the other hand, you have highly educated baby boomers who question everything and walk into the hospital with their ten-page birthing plan when they go into labor. The key is to find the physician who meets your needs.

Another consideration when choosing a physician is staffing coverage for his/her practice on their days off. Find out if other physicians in the group will see you or the name or names of other area physicians who can attend to you if you should be ill or injured during your physician's absence.

Another consideration is where a surgeon performs his surgery. Is it performed at a local hospital or in a freestanding surgical facility? A local hospital is preferred if the person has a complicated medical history. There are more resources available if any complications develop during a procedure or surgery. There are many freestanding surgical facilities. Some surgeons may jointly own the off-hospital-site surgical centers. They are most likely to steer you to this facility for surgery. This arrangement has many positive benefits for the surgeon. He has more accessible time in an operating room and thereby can perform more surgeries. You should check with your state to determine if this facility is licensed, inspected and accredited by JACHO (The Joint Commission). It should meet the same standards as those in a hospital operating room. In some states, mini-surgical centers are located in strip malls. Cosmetic surgeries are performed in these unlicensed facilities. In my home state, a large, well-known, privately owned surgical facility was determined to be sterilizing "one-time" single-use surgical instruments and reusing them on several patients. The surgical instruments were meant to be used once and thrown away.

You may wonder why this would occur? It saves money for the owners and partners of the surgical center who may in fact be the surgeons themselves. One of the surgeons in the group refused to re-use sterilized one-time-use instruments because he felt using instruments that may become dull over time with repeated use could compromise his surgery. The facility was also reprimanded for failing to follow proper procedures in administering anesthesia. According to a copy of the State's Complaint/Incident Investigation Report, this facility "failed to follow proper procedures in administering anesthesia because an anesthesiologist left a patient unattended during the administration of anesthesia to check on other patients." (69) They were cited by the Department of Public Health.

A large hospital conducts its own checks and balances to assure quality medical care. Most hospitals will not allow non-certified surgeons to utilize their facilities. If complications do arise and your surgery was performed at a hospital, you can always go back to the hospital, at any hour, on any given day, for any problems and the medical staff will have immediate access to all the records of your surgery to enable them to treat you more effectively.

When choosing a physician, others may want to consider location and time of office hours. If it is difficult for you to travel, you may want to seek medical care close to your home. For others, the ease of getting appointments, whether it be weekends or evening appointments may be the deciding factor as to where to seek medical care.

Another consideration is your physician's age and knowledge. A study done by Harvard Medical School discovered that doctors who had been out of medical school for more than 20 years were up to 48% less likely to stay up to date on developments in their fields. (70) Of course this is not true for all doctors. Many keep abreast in their fields through medical journals and medical conferences. But if your physician seems not to know about the latest treatments or studies it may be time for a change.

A physician is not required to take the tests that allow him to be board certified in his area of specialty. He can still practice medicine without taking or even passing his board certification. However, he will likely be most up to date on current treatments and therapies if he is board certified. Board certification in a specialty varies with some having to be retested every seven years.

Ask hospital nurses who they would send their relative to if they needed a physician. Most will give you an honest answer. They see physicians and how they perform under stress, how they interact with patients and families, their skills and how they interact with staff. I had the unpleasant and uncomfortable experience of overhearing a physician berating his staff and making derogatory statements about his previous patients, while I waited in an examination room for an ophthalmologist. Needless to say, this kind of situation made me uncomfortable and I did not return to this particular ophthalmologist again.

Chapter 22

SEEKING MEDICAL CARE/SURGERY OUTSIDE THE UNITED STATES

"America's health care system is second only to Japan...Canada, Sweden, Great Britain, ... well, all of Europe. But you can thank your lucky stars we don't live in Paraguay." - Dan Castellaneta

The field of cosmetic or plastic surgery has grown tremendously in the past decade. Everyone wants to look his or her best at almost any cost. Many Americans are traveling to foreign countries for cosmetic surgeries at a fraction of the cost of that in the United States. Most insurance companies will not pay for cosmetic surgery. The costs are high. U.S. citizens may find themselves in Brazil, Mexico, Europe or elsewhere to get a facelift, breast enhancement or liposuction.

The problems that are arising are the lack of proper training (this can also occur in the United States) or proper facilities that people are going to for these procedures. The problem is growing as foreign companies advertise on the Internet and offer exclusive hotel packages when you fly to their country for surgery. They offer recovery in a spa-like atmosphere.

You most likely have no recourse for a botched surgery or one followed by complications in a foreign country. These countries do not have the same judicial systems in place. You are literally playing a game of Russian roulette with your life by going out of the country to save some money. You have no assurance that the person performing your surgery is a qualified surgeon. In fact, there have been cases where people were posing as surgeons in foreign countries and were anything but a surgeon.

A reputable cosmetic surgeon should be accredited by the American Society of Plastic Surgeons. They maintain a Web site at www.plasticsurgery.org. You are able to search for an accredited physician by name, location or zip code.

I have read in magazines, newspapers and seen on television case after case of cosmetic surgery that did not go as planned which led to permanent disfigurement and/or death.

Of course, there are consumers who just use poor judgment when choosing the who and where of health care. In Woburn, Massachusetts, in March 2008, a Brazilian physician, who was not licensed to practice in the United States, performed liposuction on a woman on a massage table in a basement. The 24-year-old woman died during the procedure. The physician was sentenced to two to three years in prison for his role in the death. (71) One can only speculate the reasons this woman chose to allow this physician to perform any procedure on her.

There are many more similar cases. I'm sure if the families of these people or the victims themselves could turn back the clock, they would have chosen differently.

U.S. citizens have also attempted to procure organs in foreign countries where they are able to buy a kidney. The need for donor hearts, kidneys, liver, corneas and even bone marrow continues to rise as the field of transplantation continues to improve with many successes. The buying and selling of organs in foreign countries are often brokered through a third party. Many of the poor people are persuaded to sell a kidney only to receive only a fraction of the money they were promised after medical expenses and broker fees are paid. There is often little or no follow-up care for these people after the surgery is done. Such sale of organs is illegal in the United States and the United Kingdom where waiting lists for cadaver organs is high and lists continues to grow. This new phenomena is being referred to as "transplant tourism."

Some countries like the Philippines recognize the need and have attempted to meet the needs of all involved head-on. The government promises long term economic support and medical care for the donors rather than an upfront cash incentive. It's aimed at eliminating the black market in human organs, which often exploits poverty stricken donors.

Chapter 23

SECOND OPINIONS

"Faith is taking the first step even when you don't see the whole staircase." -- Martin Luther King Jr.

There are many reasons for consulting another physician or surgeon for a second opinion.

Some of them may include:

- Whenever non-emergency surgery is advised;
- When a medical condition does not appear to be improving despite treatment;
- A reoccurrence of a medical condition after treatment;
- Persistent symptoms despite treatment;
- Many treatment options are available and you are unclear which is best for your condition;
- You have been advised that there are no further treatments available for your condition; or
- You have many unanswered questions.

Most health care insurance carriers will allow for a second opinion. It makes good financial sense. If a surgeon recommends surgery that will cost thousands of dollars and the problem can be treated medically in a less costly manner, the insurance company can save thousands of dollars all for the cost of the second opinion. HMOs may be less likely to cover the cost of a second opinion.

Second opinions are common when a physician/surgeon suggests surgery for an ailment. Yet, it is estimated that half of Americans don't get a second opinion. Prevention Health Magazine reported, "Nearly 2.5 million people go under the knife unnecessarily, often with devastating consequences." The same article goes on to say, "one study showed that when patients and doctors share the decision making, rates of surgery drop by as much as 44%."(72)

The challenge arises of where to seek the second opinion. You can ask the first physician and surgeon for a recommendation, however, they may send you to a colleague who is less likely to contradict a friend. You can try to find a large university hospital or physician that specializes in your condition and is not associated with your physician. You will need to take your insurance plan into consideration unless you are willing to self-pay for the second opinion.

As I mentioned previously, a relative had two diverse opinions from two separate surgeons. Of course, the dilemma then is whose opinion do you trust, allow and follow. It may be that both are correct and that there would be no further injury or serious consequences if surgery were delayed. However, in a stressful situation, a second opinion may add more confusion to the final decision. Remember that the final decision is always up to the patient. That decision may be based on fear, confusion, denial or a realm of other issues. It is often more comfortable to take the easy road to avoid an unpleasant treatment, test or examination, but it may not be the right decision. If you tell your friends and family, they may come up with additional conflicting information as to whether they had a positive or negative outcome in a similar situation. Ultimately, a decision must be made and an informed and educated decision is usually the best. I must add that not all hospitals are created equal. One facility may have an outstanding birthing center, with high-risk perinatologists and neonatologists working there. This does not guarantee that they have an outstanding cardiac facility in which you should have your open-heart surgery. You may need to expand your horizons to get the best care in different locations for different medical conditions.

The same can be said for emergency room care. A 2007 CDC (Centers for Disease Control) report indicated emergency department visits are up 20 percent over the last ten years and the number of emergency departments available to treat these patients has dropped by 9% during the same period. (73) Depending on the hospital and location, some may only employ one emergency physician per shift. They may utilize an "on-call" system for necessary specialists. This can result in a timely delay in critical treatment. So check out local hospitals in your area, if you have a choice, to best determine their physician-staffing situation regarding pediatric specialists, trauma care, cardiac, neurosurgeon and orthopedic surgeons.

Getting into a crowded emergency room for emergent care on a Friday or Saturday night can be frustrating. If in fact you do have a suspected major medical emergency, never hesitate to call 911 for an ambulance. When you arrive at the hospital emergency room in an ambulance, you will receive priority care. However, with hospital emergency rooms experiencing all-time record crowding, even those arriving by ambulance may be forced to wait. Emergency rooms use a system called "triage." Those coming in the door are quickly assessed and evaluated for the acuity of their illness or injury. The people with the most acute illness or injury are given priority status to be examined and treated first.

Beyond getting priority care at an emergency room, calling an ambulance may be the wiser choice when you or a loved one needs immediate medical help. One of my relatives had a cardiac pacemaker in place, experienced chest pain in the middle of the night. He called his two elderly siblings to take him to the emergency room. They, of course, drove him in the car to the nearest emergency room, which was 10 miles away. Fortunately, all turned out well but the potential for a catastrophic event was in place. Neither the driver nor the passenger knew CPR. Had the person experienced a life threatening heart arrhythmia or heart attack, the outcome could have been drastically different. I advised all involved that the next time an ambulance needed to be called. Minutes can make the difference between life and death. Ambulances can be at our side usually in a matter of minutes and are staffed by Emergency Medical Technicians with the training and equipment to evaluate, stabilize and treat those who are ill or injured.

A friend of mine, who is a Registered Nurse, works at the same local hospital that I had worked at for many years. When her son sustained a cut on his face that required sutures she took him to the Emergency room. Unfortunately, it occurred on a Friday night when emergency rooms are usually quite busy. My friend was made to wait in the emergency waiting room for several hours before a physician could see her son. She frequently checked with the nurses and had no luck expediting his care. Finally, they were called in and she was told that her son needed sutures. My friend asked that a plastic surgeon be called because the laceration was on the face. She was told that there was none available. Only after telling the staff that she was a nurse at the very same hospital and threatening to go to another hospital was a plastic surgeon called. The plastic surgeon came in, was very kind to her son, but asked, "Why didn't they call me a few hours ago before I went to bed?"

In late summer of 2007, I received a phone call from a family member who was told she needed major surgery. She had already chosen a general surgeon known by her group of friends, across the state from where her close family lived. The hospital where the surgeon practiced was a small community hospital. When I researched the surgeon on the State Medical Examining Board. I uncovered some unflattering news about him. The allegations included (but not limited to):

He failed to:

-provide rapid and appropriate preoperative treatment and care;

- use a proper suction drain;

- adequately monitor a patient's post-operative condition;

 - employ proper diagnostic measures and tools in evaluating and monitoring the patient's post-operative condition;

- discover an acute hemorrhage from the surgical site;

- adequately maintain the patient's medical condition and/or

- failed to take and keep full and adequate medical records. (74)

The patient referred to in those allegations died and the physician was ordered to pay a civil penalty of less than $10,000.

My family member who had chosen this surgeon was offered his name from several close friends. I went to visit her and offer my assistance with appointments with a surgeon, her care and follow-up. I told her I was willing to do this, but knew nothing about her medications, her medical history, the names of her out-of-state doctors and so many other issues. We immediately sat down and started a notebook with all the relevant information. At least some-one would know where to get the answers if she was unable to give them. I then told her that I preferred that she see a vascular surgeon (as opposed to the general surgeon) and went to a hospital much larger than the small one across the state, far from her family. Fortunately, I took her to a surgeon for a second opinion who stated that she did not need the surgery!

Another article I read detailed the health of a young 47-year-old woman who experienced sudden exhaustion. Believing that her problems were a respiratory infection, her physician placed her on antibiotics. Several weeks later, her symptoms had not resolved. Eventually, it was determined that she needed a heart valve replacement. She traveled to a larger medical center away from her home for the surgery. Six weeks after the heart valve replacement, she was still experiencing the same symptoms as previously. She made an appointment with a local cardiologist for a second opinion. It was discovered that the heart valve that had been replaced was the incorrect size. She needed another surgery, which was a success.

This woman paid attention to her body and sought additional opinions when she felt things were not right. (75)

A relative of mine knew something was wrong with her arm when she could no longer move it and was in severe pain. She saw her personal physician for months without a diagnosis and her condition deteriorated. She finally went to a local emergency room for help. Her only error was stating to the physician on call "I'm here for a second opinion." This immediately turned the physician against her. If she had stated that her arm felt numb and she was unable to move it, she hopefully would have gotten the immediate help and diagnosis that she desperately needed. Instead, her comment was met with, "We don't give second opinions here," and she was not even physically examined. She finally had to demand that her personal physician order an MRI (Magnetic Resonance Imaging). Her personal physician finally took notice of her complaints and metastatic bone cancer was found on MRI.

When my son was about five years old, I took him to an eye specialist at the urging of his pediatrician. The physician thought my son had a "lazy eye" or that the muscle that affected the normal alignment of his eyes was slightly weak. I hadn't noticed any actual difference but followed the physician's orders and scheduled an appointment. To my amazement, the eye surgeon recommended immediate surgery to "tighten" the muscle that holds the eye in alignment. He strongly suggested that this be done prior to my son entering kindergarten. He advised us that he would actually "overcorrect" this problem so that my son's eye would stay aligned as he continued to grow. You can imagine my immediate concerns, as I never even suspected that my son had a visual problem or an alignment issue. Well, I didn't take this surgeon's recommendation as the final word and immediately decided to take my son to a local children's hospital located in my state for a second opinion. The second surgeon not only did more sophisticated testing, but also stated, "There is nothing wrong with your son's eyes. They may have been "tired" on the day of the first exam with the other surgeon, but he does not need surgery." We followed up with the surgeon for several years and it has been 23 years since I was told that my son needed corrective surgery. He never had surgery, his eyes are in perfect alignment and he has 20-20 vision. I shudder to think what could have happened if I had not listened to my instincts and sought a second opinion.

I also experienced the reverse on several occasions. Sometimes an omission to diagnose is made. My son was extremely small in stature for his age group. One of my biggest concerns was the fact that he still had all his baby teeth at the age of nine years. I brought this to the attention of two different pediatricians in the medical practice where I took him. One of them actually belittled me by saying, "Stop being a nurse and be a mother." At my son's next pediatric dental appointment, the dentist actually spoke to me about concerns regarding a possible growth delay due to the fact that my son still had his baby teeth well past the age that most of his peers had lost theirs. This dentist was able to facilitate an appointment with an endocrinologist at Yale New Haven Hospital where it was confirmed that my son did in fact have a three-year growth delay. Needless to say, I found a new pediatric group.

I was fortunate to have a good health insurance program that has covered my expenses regarding second opinions. Not everyone is as fortunate.

With the advent and popularity of the Internet, many can find a multitude of forums, health topics, support message boards and other information relating to illnesses. Opinions can vary widely. I don't advise getting all your health information from the Internet. Message boards can be a great tool for coping and networking with others who suffer from similar problems or illnesses. However, as I have warned previously, everyone is an individual and may respond differently to treatments and medications. Many Internet messaging and support boards will have a medical advisor, but they are cautious not to give specific treatment regimens over the Internet. The more reliable Web sites are those related to large organizations and URL's end in .com (commercial,) .edu (educational institution), .gov (government) or .org (organization). A URL address does not guarantee authentic information on a Web site. Dishonest people are able to make a Web site look authentic when in reality it is not.

Caution is always advised when using the Internet and should never substitute for a visit with your physician.

A new avenue for second opinions has come to light with the introduction of Electronic Second Opinions. One that came to my attention recently was the Cleveland Clinic and Partner's Center for Connected Health. (They are affiliated with Harvard Medical School.) See the Resources Information section at the end of this book for Web site address.

I am sure that the availability of electronic second opinions will increase in the next few years. Of course, there are limitations with this system. The physician never actually sees the patient in person and does not get to perform a hands-on physical assessment. However, it may have potential when reviewing laboratory or pathology reports in correlation to a detailed medical history. Registration is required to use these services and some nominal fees may be charged. Because this method is relatively new, it is uncertain if your insurance company will cover these second opinions. The cost can range up to several hundred dollars for an opinion. A relative did initiate a second opinion consultation with the Cleveland Clinic and Blue Cross of Connecticut agreed to pay for it.

It is always good to seek a second opinion when your surgeon advises non-emergency surgery. Some health plans may dictate that a second opinion is necessary. Ask your physician or surgeon for an alternate way to treat the condition without surgery. Another important question to ask is how many times a year a surgeon performs a specific surgery and how many times it is performed in the hospital that he utilizes. Statistically, time has shown that the more times a surgeon has done a procedure, the better the outcome. Of course, this carries no guarantees, but experience does count. You want a surgeon and hospital that have been doing the procedure at a high rate for many years, with a majority of positive outcomes. See chapter 23 - Second Opinions.

Another instance when a second opinion may be needed is when your health condition is not improving over time. A family member recently had a skin rash for three months, and it was not clearing up despite antibiotics and ointments. The pediatrician kept advocating a wait-and-see approach, despite the child's discomfort. Finally, a call for a second opinion was made and a correct diagnosis was made after skin cultures were performed. The entire process took four months to get a correct diagnosis.

Sometimes, a third opinion may be necessary. A good friend was seriously injured in an automobile accident. The impact was so severe that the man crushed the steering wheel with his chest. He was hospitalized for several days and X-rays were taken. He went home to recuperate and was still having severe chest pain that had not gotten any better. He went back to his personal physician and complained about the pain. The physician's response was, "You should get down on your knees and be thankful you are alive." The second physician he saw told him that he would give him another two weeks off from work, but that would be all. The physician didn't want to get in trouble with the patient's employer. This physician also made a comment to the wife that alluded that her husband was a "gold digger." A third opinion was sought, from a concerned physician who took the time to track down the original X-rays, only to discover a crack in the sternum (a bone in the middle upper portion of the chest).

Usually enlisting the aid of your physician to get you an appointment for a second opinion will speed up the waiting process but this is not always so. Ask your physician if he can assist you in the appointment making process. Your physician can also assist you by supplying the consulting physician with copies of laboratory test results, medical records, x-ray or other films and background information that he or she feels is relevant to your case.

Some people will simply go for a second opinion without telling the first physician. This is usually a mistake. It is usually best to bring all previous testing results to the second physician or surgeon. Your physician or surgeon should be happy to assist you in obtaining the best second opinion available. Valuable time and money can be wasted by not telling the second physician that you have already had previous testing done and the results. Your health insurance carrier may not cover testing the second time around. Of course, there is always the chance that you may get two completely differing opinions and walk out more confused than ever. You can always go back to the first physician and discuss your options again and hopefully come up with a mutually agreed upon treatment plan.

Look for a second opinion at a large university research and teaching hospital if possible. The chances are that new treatments and therapies may be available at large hospitals that have not gotten to your local physician or surgeon yet. Some of these facilities will also present your "case" before a board of specialists thereby rendering the opinions and recommendations of many physicians.

As I mentioned previously, check if your second opinion physician/surgeon is board certified in the area of expertise that you require. The American Board of Medical Specialties can be found at www.abms.org.

Chapter 24

BETTER DOCTOR/PATIENT RELATIONSHIPS

"A doctor who cannot take a good history and a patient who cannot give one are in danger of giving and receiving bad treatment." - Author Unknown

I have previously discussed how you can be a better informed and better-prepared patient.

A good physician will have good physical assessment skills and be a good communicator. It may sound trivial, but scheduling a yearly physical exam with your physician is a great way to build your relationship with your physician. Your physician has scheduled the time - usually longer than "sick" visits - and can use this time to see you when you are well. It is estimated that only 72% of us schedule an annual visit. According to an article published in Woman's Day Magazine in February 2008, reasons most given for not having an annual check-up include:

- money;

- time;
- fear;
- ease about discussing personal issues - 38%;
- cost of prescriptions - 53% stated that they would forgo a prescribed medication due to cost; and
- fear of a diagnosis of cancer, with 28% of Americans concerned about it. (76)

It makes sense if we go to our personal physician on a regular basis and communicate any changes in our bodies. Cancer or any other health issue may be diagnosed sooner and therefore have better outcomes. An annual physical is an invaluable tool to help your physician determine what tests, vaccines and treatments you need for long-standing health issues. During "ill" appointments, he/she will only be focusing on the issue that brought you in.

I previously discussed many aspects of saving money on prescriptions in Chapter 14. Talking with your physician about your medication and difficulty with costs can be beneficial. If a prescription is too costly, there may be other medications that have the desired effect at a lower cost. You can ask the pharmacist who is familiar with medications and costs, but it is ultimately up to the physician to change a medication once it has been ordered. Physicians also have access to professional samples. These are medications that pharmaceutical representatives bring to physician offices in order to educate them and encourage them to prescribe them in the scope of their practice. These are of limited supply and you will not be allowed to get all your medications free from the doctor's office. If, however, a medication is prescribed for a short term, ask your physician if he has any professional samples. This is also a good trial if you are unsure if you will be able to tolerate a new prescription. If you try the professional samples and have no problem, you can then fill the long-term prescription.

Usually newer medications to the market are more expensive. Over time, they become generic and are marketed by other drug companies and the cost goes down. Be sure to ask your physician if there is another medication on the market that is less expensive if you pay for your own prescriptions and have no insurance coverage. Nearly 47 million Americans, or 16 percent of the population, were without health insurance in 2005 with an estimate of over 36% of seniors without prescription coverage. (77)

Chapter 25

DIFFICULT DECISIONS

"Quick decisions are unsafe decisions." - Sophocles

Medical decisions can be minor or major and can impact your health care. The reason behind your decision can depend on a variety of factors, be it fear, finances or poor understanding.

Some questions to ask your physician/surgeon may include the following:

- Do I really need this test or surgery?
- What is the expected outcome of this procedure?
- Is there any preparation for this test/procedure?
- Is there any recovery from this test/procedure?
- How many of these specific surgeries do you perform a year? The rule of thumb here is the more the better. You want a surgeon who is experienced with the procedure that you require.

- Will you have another doctor assisting you in the operating room? Surgeons do not operate alone. Most surgeons utilize surgical residents if the surgery is performed in a "teaching hospital." This means that the hospital that your are using has a Physician Residency Program that has "student doctors" on staff for a period of usually four years so that they can learn the specifics of a certain field of medicine. These are "doctors in training" that I discussed earlier in the book. Depending on what year the resident is in his/her training will play a role in how involved he is with your actual surgery. Note that new residents come to the hospital July 1st of each calendar year. You do have a right to "no residents" while in the hospital or during the surgery if you have private insurance that pays for your hospitalization. However, if you are having a complex surgery, your surgeon needs to know prior to your day of surgery if you plan to use "no residents" as he may need to make additional arrangements to get another surgeon in for the operation. The majority of patients allow surgical residents in to assist their surgeon so it is not a large issue. In addition, there will be a scrub nurse in the operating room, (she hands the surgeon his instruments during the operation), a circulating nurse, (she documents and retrieves any items needed), the anesthesiologist, (he monitors your vital signs and administers the medication to make you "sleep" during your surgery).

During surgery, the resident doctor acts as extended eyes and hands for the surgeons (the attending) in the hospital. You will actually be seen by more doctors by allowing the residents in to see you. Because they are less experienced, they are apt to be more thorough.

- Ask what the alternatives of your treatment or care may be. Some physicians may not mention these unless asked.

With any major illness or trauma, difficult decisions may have to be made. In most instances, you will be asked to make a medical decision on behalf of yourself or family member. Some doctors will make it appear that you have no choice in the matter, but in reality you do have a choice. I cautioned you earlier, however, to use your "right to refuse" with caution.

In a real life-or-death situation, the physician will simply tell you in a hurried fashion what he needs to do to attempt to save the life of a loved one. There may not be time for informed decisions in this situation.

However, a new cancer diagnosis or major illness can create quite a challenge. You can be hit from all sides, while you are emotionally devastated and be asked to make lifesaving decisions. The best way to help yourself or your loved one is to be informed.

Ask questions, take notes and get a second opinion. Ultimately, the final decisions regarding your treatment are up to you. You must be willing to accept that medicine is not an exact science. You can visit two different physicians and get two opposite opinions, which can lead to more confusion. If you have gotten two different opinions from two surgeons you can refer back to your primary care physician for guidance if you know him/her well and respect their judgment. You might even ask them what they would do if this were their spouse with this diagnosis.

You can attempt to educate yourself by going to your local library, which should have a reference section on medical books. These may be difficult to understand and of course you can't ask the book any questions.

You can ask the physician/surgeon for printed literature to take home and read on the topic. When you are home in a relaxed, quiet environment, you may be able to read and understand the literature a little better.

You can go on the Internet. Please use caution. There are many people who post their medical experiences online, be it good or bad. However, they are not you, and each person is an individual with different risk factors. Try to stick to sites that are sponsored by well known organizations, such as the American Cancer Society. These organizations can be a wonderful resource for newly diagnosed patients.

An exciting new trend is the use of Cancer Coaches. The American Cancer Society has begun providing cancer coaches, or patient advocates, trained volunteers or paid coaches to help navigate the confusing time after a patient first receives a diagnosis of cancer. A Cancer Coach can provide information that is hopefully more reliable and less confusing than well-intentioned family and friends. The National Breast Cancer Coalition also trains coaches and many coaches are starting to appear in large teaching hospitals. Unfortunately, the need for coaches currently surpass their numbers, but you can call the American Cancer Society, The National Breast Cancer Coalition, or your local teaching hospital for references. Ultimately, they will provide you with current support and information, but the final decision regarding your specific needs are between you and your physician/surgeon.

Chapter 26

A BIG FIX FOR HEALTHCARE
& HEALTHCARE INSURANCE

"If you are too smart to pay the doctor, you had better be too smart to get ill." -   African Proverb

Our health may be one of the biggest things in life that we take for granted until it is threatened. Most of us are too busy with our daily lives to consider the dire costs that one major accident or illness can incur.   I know family members who were self employed and had young children. They felt that the private pay premiums were too expensive and opted not to pay, simply going without health insurance. The quote I heard most was, "we're all healthy here." When it was time for required school physical examinations - "well" visits as they are referred to - the family would simply negotiate the cost with the physician's office when the bill came. Many physician offices will negotiate their fees for "private pay" patients.   Many will charge the medical insurance or Medicare a larger fee, as they know that only a percentage or agreed-upon amount will actually be paid.

The truth of the matter is, whether you can afford health insurance or not, the cost of one major medical event, either illness or accident, can be staggering. Whether or not you have insurance may even affect how soon you are treated and how much treatment you will receive. A report from the National Academies Institute of Medicine, states the uninsured are about 1.4 times more likely to die prematurely due to lack of health insurance. Uninsured patients with colon or breast cancer face up to a 50 percent greater chance of dying than patients with private coverage. (78)

Those who are fortunate to be employed may have a substantial health insurance plan, with contributions made by both the employer and the employee. If your employer offers group coverage, you have a right under Federal Law to be enrolled in the plan. Your coverage and contributions will vary based of the number of actual plans offered by the employer. Each employer holds "open enrollment" on an annual basis. New literature is printed with specific coverage costs regarding, co-pays, limitations and exclusions, lifetime maximums, pharmacy, dental or eye care packages. Obtain a copy of this information yearly and review it carefully. Never assume that the plan that you had the previous year will continue, "as is." If you or someone in your family is frequently at the physician's office, you may want to opt for a higher co-pay but better coverage for the frequent office visits. Over the years, most of us have seen these contributions from our paychecks increase and higher co-pays to see our physicians. A high deductible and 20% co-pay for services can add hundreds of dollars of savings over the course of a year, and save you from potential financial ruin in the event of a catastrophic illness.

Some large corporations and businesses even allow incentives for losing weight, exercising and smoking cessation classes. Check with your place of employment and see if they offer these. If not, see if they are willing to consider it.

Another newer option are Flexible Health Savings Plans. These programs were initiated in 1979, with the Health Reimbursement option coming onto the scene in 2002. These programs are offered by employers to allow employees to pay for certain health care costs or dependent expenses before being taxed on the income.

There are several recognized Flexible Spending Accounts. They appear to still be evolving and gaining publicity and popularity. They include the Health Care Flexible Spending Account, the Limited Expense Health Care Flexible Spending Account and the Dependent Care Flexible Spending Account. Enrollment in these plans is voluntary and is done through your employer on an annual basis, similar to your open enrollment insurance plan. You need to know that you have to estimate your costs wisely as you stand to lose money that has not been used to pay for health care after a period of 14 1/2 months. This is called the "use it or lose it" rule. (79). I would advise anyone interested in one of these plans to sit down with their employer's health insurance specialist prior to investing in this program to understand what exactly is covered and what is not, to see if it will benefit you.

The U.S. Department of Labor, Bureau of Labor Statistics has detailed information regarding this program on their Web site at: www.bls.gov. This program is not portable to a new job. You must remain at the same employer to access your Flexible Spending Account.

A Health Savings Account may be a better option for some. Under this plan, established in 2003, money is set-aside in a savings account, prior to taxes, to enable the individual to pay for medical costs now and in the future. Money can be added up until the age of 65 years. After that, money can be withdrawn for any purpose. There are still limitations to this program. Some of the key ones include: the individual can NOT be covered by any other health insurance, NOT enrolled in Medicare and the person contributing can NOT be claimed as a dependent on any other person's tax return. You can obtain detailed information about a Health Savings Account from the United States Treasury Department. (80)

The Internal Revenue Service also places maximum caps on Health Savings Accounts. In other words, they limit the amount of money that an individual can place into the account for family health expenses. A Health Savings Account can be taken with you to a new job at a different employer.

Many families are not able to make these payments and simply lack health care insurance. Overall, 47 million people lacked health insurance in 2006, the census numbers showed, up from 44.8 million in 2005. The percentage of the U.S. population lacking health insurance in 2006 rose to 15.8%, the highest level since 1998. In 2005, 15.3% were uninsured. (81)

Many long-term employees who had worked for the same company for over 25 years assumed they would have employee medical insurance coverage when they retired. An alarming new trend is the fact that many were not covered as anticipated. These numbers are expected to rise in the future. Some companies had written contracts that stated they would be covered, but over time, companies closed, went bankrupt, left the country for cheaper labor and left their longtime devoted employees holding the bag.

Some employees may find themselves putting off the age of retirement until they are sure they will be covered by Medicare and Social Security. However, as I have discussed earlier, these cannot be counted on to cover extensive medical costs and a company can change its health care policies at any time. More and more Americans are finding themselves taking out a second mortgage or digging into their retirement funds to pay for a single catastrophic health event that was not fully covered by insurance. It is estimated that about 50% of bankruptcies can be blamed on medical bills, most of these families being middle class. (82) This predicament can happen to anyone.

Many state, federal and military employees are finding themselves with the same health care coverage issues. The private sector is not alone. Considering your options during your employment years may benefit you in the future. You may want to consider a healthier lifestyle now, before long-term damage is done, to help allay medical costs in your retirement years. Also if you utilize your health insurance plan now to get regular health checkups, you may be able to prevent or delay serious health issues in the future.

Investigate your health care coverage prior to retirement and find out if you are eligible for COBRA (Consolidated Omnibus Budget Reconciliation Act of 1985) benefits. COBRA health care coverage allows for you to keep your current medical insurance health plan for a limited period of time after you have left your current employment, with you paying the total premium up to 102 %.

According to the United States Department of Labor, if you lose or leave your job, or if another event occurs that would cause you to lose coverage under an employer's group health plan, you may have the right to COBRA benefits.

There are a number of considerations you should take into account, including:

- whether other group health coverage -- such as coverage under another employer's plan -- is available;
- whether any other available health coverage would exclude benefits for a medical condition that you or a family member has;
- when you will have the right to enroll in the other coverage;
- the cost, scope and level of COBRA coverage compared with that of any other available group coverage or individual health coverage; and
- whether a guaranteed right to buy individual health coverage is important to you. (83)

If paying your COBRA benefits is important to you and you cannot afford to make the premium payments due to unemployment, you may want to check if you can use your IRA (Individual Retirement Account) for payment without penalty.

One of the positive things that resulted from HIPAA (The Health Insurance Portability and Accountability) when it became law in 1996, was the protection of your rights to health insurance when you lose your job or change your job.

Some private insurers are offering short-term coverage to bridge the transition between employers. Check with several insurance companies in your area to determine if they offer such a policy. The cost may be reasonable as they are offering the policy for a short period of time and feel their exposure to costly payouts is limited.

Title I of HIPAA regulates the availability and breadth of group and individual health insurance plans. It amends both the Employee Retirement Income Security Act and the Public Health Service Act. Title I prohibits any group health plan from creating eligibility rules or assessing premiums for individuals in the plan based on health status, medical history, genetic information or disability. This does not apply to private individual insurance.

Title I also limits restrictions that a group health plan can place on benefits for preexisting conditions. Group health plans may refuse to provide benefits relating to preexisting conditions for a period of 12 months after enrollment in the plan or 18 months in the case of late enrollment. However, individuals may reduce this exclusion period if they had health insurance prior to enrolling in the plan. Title I allows individuals to reduce the exclusion period by the amount of time that they had "creditable coverage" prior to enrolling in the plan and after any "significant breaks" in coverage. "Creditable coverage" is defined quite broadly and includes nearly all group and individual health plans, including Medicare and Medicaid. A "significant break" in coverage is defined as any 63-day period without any creditable coverage. (84)

Those who have no health care insurance and little or no money for health care can get medical care through the Bureau of Primary Health. The Department of Human Resources funds primary care facilities across the nation for at-risk communities with high numbers of people in need of medical help with little or no financial resources. A list of facilities can be accessed by state on their Web site at: http://ask.hrsa.gov/pc/.

The State of Connecticut began accepting applications in July 2008 for a new Charter Oak Health Plan. It is only being offered to an estimated 5 or 6% uninsured residents of Connecticut. The program offers low state-subsidized premiums for basic health care including primary care and maternity care. This program accepts those with preexisting conditions. Getting hospitals to participate in the Charter Oak Health Plan was slower than initially expected, but the numbers of participating hospitals has continued to grow. According to Connecticut Governor, M. Jodi Rell's office, within the first two weeks of the Charter Oak Health plan, there were over 7,000 phone calls from people that were interested in learning more about the program. There were 1,950 enrollments in the plan in the first two weeks. Clearly the need for such a program is there. Another proposed plan in Connecticut is the ConnPACE Plus program. This program is now being considered to allow senior citizens to save nearly $1,160 a year on Medicare premiums and co-pays on prescription medications. Due to the current budget constraints of the state, this initiative is on hold.

HIPAA rules can differ from state to state, so it is important to check your locale for specific information. Anyone with a preexisting medical condition may be eligible for a "High Risk Pool" similar to those offered for automotive drivers with a poor driving history record. Higher premiums may be paid for a period of time, however, at least some coverage will be afforded.

Also, don't forget to keep copies of medical bills and prescriptions that you paid for yourself to apply toward your income tax as an itemized deduction.

Having large outstanding medical bills that you can't afford to pay can also affect your credit report. In years past, single physician practices or local hospitals handled their own billing and debt collection. That has changed in the past ten years. Physician offices and hospitals are taking a much more aggressive approach to getting paid by hiring debt-collection agencies to handle any outstanding debts after a brief attempt to collect from the consumer. These companies will quickly add these negative debts to your credit report.

The real solution for health insurance may be to open the market with more healthcare insurance companies that allow for purchasing insurance across state lines and making it portable with any job. More competition in the insurance market could possibly lead to lower premiums and the ability to carry the same insurance with you irrespective of where you work much like our home and auto insurance policies.

Chapter 27

GETTING THE CARE YOU NEED

"If a free society cannot help the many who are poor, it cannot save the few who are rich."
John F. Kennedy, inaugural address, January 20, 1961

For those without health care insurance, Medicare may be the answer if you fit the criteria. Medicare is a health insurance program for people age 65 or older, some disabled people under age 65, and people of all ages with End-Stage Renal Disease (permanent kidney failure treated with dialysis or a transplant). (85) Even those with Medicare coverage over age 65 may want to consider a private-pay supplemental insurance plan to cover other medical care if they can afford it.

Most states also provide health insurance for children whose parents cannot afford health care coverage for their dependents. Coverage is usually limited to minor age children with specific household income requirements. In Connecticut, we utilize the

HUSKY Plan, under the direction of the State of Connecticut, Department of Social Services. Check with your state for specific enrollment requirements. The government has an international Web site at www.Insurekidsnow.net. (86) Another government-sponsored program is set up through the Department of Health and Human Services. By using their Web site, www.hrsa.gov, you can click on "Find Help, Health Care regardless of your ability to pay." Once there, simply put in a city and state and you will be directed to many health care facilities that will treat you at low or no cost.

One group of people who are struggling for adequate health insurance coverage are young men and women between the ages of 19 and 29 years. In 2005, 29.3 percent of this group did not have health insurance, a jump of 2.2 million since 2000. (87) This number is expected to rise. Many are covered on their parents' health insurance policies until age 19. If they continue on to college as a full-time student, they most likely will be covered until about the age of 23, although this can vary depending on the state and the individual policy. For those not attending college full-time, health insurance benefits may cease. Unless these young adults obtain full-time employment, which includes medical benefits, they may find themselves in a dire financial situation in the case of serious illness or injury. Some states are passing new laws to allow young adults to remain on a parent's policy well into their mid 20's.

Having no health insurance does not mean you should forego preventative health care or treatment. Most states have outreach programs where women can obtain low-cost or free mammograms, pap smears or other testing. Women with low income and no health insurance, aged 18 to 64, are eligible for free mammograms and cervical cancer screenings. All 50 states provide these services through the National Breast and Cervical Cancer Early Detection Program.

Medical teaching schools and hospitals can be invaluable to low-income families that need care. Various clinics are held and medical students, under the auspices of their instructors, provide treatment. The wait time may be a little longer to get in to see the doctor, but excellent medical care can be found.

Hospitals also offer free health screenings, usually specific to prostate, breast, colorectal, blood pressure or blood glucose at little or no cost. They are usually held on specific dates with pre-registration being necessary. Just call your local hospital or ask your physician's office for assistance. Many newspapers advertise these health-screening events well in advance.

Some hospitals are also associated with a dental school. Again, you may have to wait for an appointment, but the care you receive is under the student and his attending instructor. No treatment is done without the instructor's consent. The amount of time from start to finish may take longer, but the end result should be the same as if you went to a private dentist.

Some dental and health clinics will present you with a written estimate for any medical or dental work that you require before you begin treatment. Some may expect your co-pay up front before any treatment is started. Determine what your insurance carrier will cover and what you will be expected to pay. Also ask the treating physician to negotiate fees or charges. This is more apt to be a viable solution if the physician owns the practice. Those who work in a large institution may have no control over the billing process. Be sure to ask to speak to a financial consultant at the institution if you anticipate difficulty paying your bill. Remember that you may be able to get similar treatment or care at another facility, possibly at a reduced rate. Be sure to shop around if money is an issue. Some outpatient testing may be cheaper if it is performed as an inpatient in the hospital. You will have to do a little investigating and compare.

Freestanding surgical centers have sprung up all over the United States in the past several years. These facilities are staffed and equipped to perform minor surgical procedures under the care of a surgeon and anesthesiologist and are often referred to as ambulatory or outpatient surgical centers. Some are owned and managed by local hospitals and some are owned by groups of physicians and anesthesiologists. Having your "minor" surgical procedure done in one of these centers can save money when compared to a hospital operating room. You need to check if the facility is accredited, preferably by JCAHO (The Joint Commission), and the credentials of those who will be administering your anesthesia and performing your surgical procedure are properly trained and licensed to do so. Most of the freestanding surgical centers tend to be very efficient, and surgeries do not get "bumped" due to emergency surgeries. So schedules appear to be more closely adhered to.

If you have a history of major medical problems, a freestanding surgical center may not be the best option for you. If a major medical complication occurs during your procedure, you may have to be transferred to a hospital and actual time can be lost in getting the best medical care. A major local hospital has a variety of specialists available to treat any possible complication. Also, if a complication arises at a freestanding surgical center, there is no hospital bed to be admitted to overnight for closer monitoring and observation.

Even psychiatric assistance can be found at psychology clinics on a sliding scale. Check with a local, large university teaching hospital for resources. The Mental Health Association, Inc. sponsors a free annual National Depression Screening Day in the month of October. Check their Web site (available in the Resources Information in the back of this book) for dates and locations.

Planned Parenthood can provide women with yearly gynecological exams at little or no cost. Free mammograms can be scheduled through the American Cancer Society, the National Cancer Institute or the American Breast Cancer Foundation. See contact information in the back of the book under Resources Information.

The Lions Clubs of America can provide eye examinations and eyeglasses for those in need. Some optometrists and other organizations offer free eye exams for those who cannot pay. Optometry Schools across the United States also offer sliding scale charges for comprehensive eye exams. If you want to save money on glasses, have your optometrist give you a written prescription of your eyeglass strength. Inexpensive reading glasses can be purchased at most local pharmacies and chain stores with various prescriptions. Another option is to find a name brand glasses frame at your local optometrist and try them on. Then go to a large warehouse store, Ebay or search for an Internet retailer that sells the same brand.

Various other national organizations sponsor free screenings for vascular disease, memory loss, heart disease, skin cancer and asthma. See the Resources Information in the back of this book under "Free Screenings" for organizations and Web site in-formation.

In an emergency situation, hospitals will treat you in an urgent situation regardless of your ability to pay. Some hospitals are required to provide care for free, but you need to determine this before there is an actual need. Otherwise, you may find yourself being forever bothered by aggressive bill collectors.

Some automobile insurance policies offer coverage in the event of an automobile accident. For those with a comprehensive health care policy, it probably is not a wise option. However, if you have no health insurance plan, an accident medical insurance rider can help cover the cost of your injuries in the event of an accident.

Medical bills are almost always negotiable. You have to sit down with the office manager or the hospital billing financial officer to work out the details of your payment schedule or for reduction in costs but it can be well worth your time and effort.

In emergency situations, you may find that your care was provided for by an "in-network" physician, however, your anesthesia, pathologist and a multitude of other "behind-the-scenes" specialists are not. I saw this trend in the 1980's but am glad to say, it seems less prevalent today. Most health insurers seem to recognize that we are not able to choose who provides our emergency care, reads our pathology or radiology reports, and it appears to be less of an issue.

As I discussed earlier, managed care is a frustrating system. The growth of managed care in the U.S. was spurred by the enactment of the Health Maintenance Organization Act of 1973. (88) "Managed care" is used to describe a variety of techniques intended to reduce the cost of providing health benefits, improve the quality of care and reduce unnecessary health care costs, including: economic incentives for physicians and patients to select less costly forms of care; programs for reviewing the medical necessity of specific services; increased beneficiary cost sharing; controls on inpatient admissions and lengths of stay; the establishment of cost-sharing incentives for outpatient surgery; selective contracting with healthcare providers; and the intensive management of high-cost healthcare cases. The programs may be provided in a variety of settings, such as Health Maintenance Organizations and Preferred Provider Organizations. (89)

It is estimated that the insurance companies spend millions of dollars trying to cut the costs of healthcare and physicians spend a great amount of time doing paperwork, being a patient advocate and justifying their decisions to insurance companies. Historically, reducing co-pays and changing our deductibles has not helped the consumer or the cost of healthcare one bit. David Cutler, a Harvard Economist, who served on President Clinton's Health Care Task Force, advises that we need to spend more money on "the stuff that works." His ideals portray a society that has vastly improved its health care in the past century, with modern treatments, advanced medical specialties and unsurpassed longevity. He wants to give physicians and hospitals incentives to do the things that keep patients healthy, as opposed to fighting the insurance companies for coverage. (90). Mr. Cutler believes to improve health care, we need to make it accessible to all Americans, make it easier to navigate the system and spend more money on health care. Advocates for this type of program encourage rewarding those physicians who have better outcomes with more pay. This would involve more follow-up contact with a physician and his patients to determine if they are following through with their prescribed treatment effectively and allow for earlier intervention if they are not. Many underinsured simply stop treatment (be it prescription or otherwise) due to cost.

Some large companies have already instituted such a plan. They are paying their physicians to make follow-up phone calls to patients and are seeing the results with fewer complications than those who did not receive intensive follow-up telephone contact after a physician office visit.

In 2008, Connecticut Senate Republicans discussed the idea of giving tax breaks for those who practice healthy lifestyles. "They unveiled legislation, that would allow people to deduct their out-of-pocket medical expenses, such as premiums and co-pays, from the state's personal income tax." (91) The idea is expanded by having prospective candidates meet certain criteria set by the state's health department; evaluated, tested and documented by their personal physician; and submitted with their taxes. Although this system could benefit those with health insurance, it would do nothing for those without or to make health care more accessible, according to critics.

The Connecticut Nurses' Association also took a closer look at improving access and affordability. In their report, they recommended focusing on:

- Prevention and early intervention programs;

- Community-based access – such as, Day care, schools – promoting screening, education and intervention, community-based clinics;

- Quality education across the life span - including more nursing scholarships to replace our retiring nursing workforce;

- Interdisciplinary collaboration; and

-Guarantee of full scope of practice.

The Connecticut Nurses' Association promotes wellness and preventative care, which is more cost effective than secondary care. (92)

An article written by Richard Conniff for MSN Money suggests other ways to improve health care. These include making health insurance more "portable" or movable from one job to another. With many Americans switching jobs, the health insurance plan is switched also. By keeping the insurance plan with the consumer, there may be more "long-term thinking" between the relationship of the consumer and his heath insurance provider.

Mr. Conniff also proposes that electronic charting, a fast growing industry in health care today, can improve our overall health care. A well-written computer program can red flag a test result or alert staff that necessary information is needed or in need of attention. He maintains that electronic charting can make for easier monitoring of laboratory tests. (93)

Social Security has been a hot topic for years. Baby boomers who paid into the system are concerned that they may not be able to collect when they reach the age of retirement. Health care costs are rising at a much faster rate than the income of those presently living on their Social Security income. Factor in the high cost of living in some parts of the country, with the high costs of gasoline and home heating oil and many senior citizens or disabled are already struggling to pay their bills. Not only are we increasing the numbers of baby boomers approaching retirement but they are also living longer when they reach retirement, which also strains the system.

Medicare and Medicaid were originally put in place for a small portion of poor people and have become increasingly relied upon for coverage of our aging population, including long-term institutionalized care in nursing facilities. Under federal law, one-quarter of the cost of Medicare must be covered by its premiums. This means that the cost of Medicare premiums will continue to rise.

Some exciting new changes are on the forefront. Mr. Joseph Stango, from my hometown, campaigned successfully to get federally funded long-term care provided for and paid for in the home by Medicare. His plan has been named "Money Follows the Person." This program will be funded by the Centers for Medicare & Medicaid Services for five years through grants.

Under the Money Follows the Person initiative, the federal government will provide increased Medicaid funding, reimbursing the state for 75 percent of costs (instead of the customary 50 percent) for the first year back in the community. Essentially, the enhanced federal support is a financial incentive for states to reduce reliance on expensive institutional care for Medicaid recipients. (94) As our elderly population increases and waiting lists for nursing homes continue to grow, now is the time to start looking for options and methods to take care of our aging population.

In Connecticut, the Medicaid Reform Bill proposed by Joseph Stango is moving forward. The four parts to this proposed bill are: "increase the current cap on participants in the first phase of the state's new Money Follows the Person home-care program; the "Bob Veillette Bill," to launch a 50-person pilot program to offer Medicaid to home care program individuals; create Dora's Trust-use Federal Grant matching money and state savings from Money

Follows the Person; enhance financial support for the new Age and Disability Resource Center." (95)

Many analysts agree with the need to provide thorough, continuing medical care in the office and home environment, as opposed to inpatient hospitalizations and nursing-home care. We need to step up our follow-up care to keep closer tabs on the patients and treatments to determine what is effective and what is not. Earlier intervention can make all the difference. Our current U.S. healthcare model is based on treatment and not prevention. We could theoretically save millions if we focus on prevention. This may initially cost more money, but will save money in the long term with reduced complications.

Chapter 28

GETTING THE BEST CARE:
YOUR RESPONSIBILITIES

"If we could give every individual the right amount of nourishment and exercise, not too little and not too much, we would have found the safest way to health. " - Hippocrates

When my mother had to have surgery, she was over-whelmed. She was an independent, intelligent woman who had limited medical knowledge, as many people who seek medical care are. She was scheduled for a surgical procedure, which completely overwhelmed her. She was sent from an internist to a surgeon to another internist, pulmonologist, cardiologist and for multiple in-depth medical tests prior to her scheduled surgery.

The medical care that my own mother received startled me. We were given little information regarding testing, no specific information regarding the impending surgery and any direct, specific questions were completely ignored by the surgeon. Questions directed at the hospital nurses regarding my mother's care were seen as intrusive and answers were nonexistent or defensive.

To prevent this from happening to you, and in order to get the best medical care, there are several things you can do.

Request a friend or advocate to accompany you to all doctor appointments. Bring the friend into the examination room, as this is where most of the physician interaction will occur, if not all of it. It is not critical that this person be a medical professional, but simply a good listener. Take notes when necessary, be sure to ask questions (devise a list prior to the appointment and write them down) and educate yourself about the impending tests or scheduled procedure as much as possible prior to the actual procedure date. You can seek further information after the appointment at your local library, another physician or an outside health professional. Remember that everyone is different, and although your neighbor may have had the same procedure, it is not reliable to compare your procedure with his or hers. Every person is an individual with specific needs and individual factors that can affect the care.

You need to communicate any relevant changes in your health in a clear, concise manner. Include such information as symptoms, when they began and how they affected your sleep, diet and activity as well as your normal routine. Be honest, and don't hold anything back. Your physician may need this information to help make a diagnosis.

To save time, bring a copy of important medical tests with you whenever possible. Many hospitals now charge for copies of your medical records if you request them through the hospital medical records department. However, you can save time by asking for a "medical release" form at the time of an actual test at a doctor's office or outpatient testing facility. Simply sign it and request that a copy be released to you when it is available. Many times, it can be mailed or you can pick up a copy several days after the test is completed. For testing that was physician ordered within the hospital, simply ask the physician for a copy for your records, as he will maintain a copy in your office chart for his records. A good physician will go over the test results with you and explain everything so that you can understand it.

Keep a folder in a safe place where other family members know where to find it. Trying to get a medical report weeks or years later is usually more difficult and can cost an exorbitant amount of money. Many hospitals now have companies that copy the medical records that a patient requests and charge dearly for these services. However, if you simply ask when you go to the physician's office it is usually given to you for free. If you are traveling, it is a good idea to bring the folder with you if you have outstanding or complicated health issues. Having the reports available for the next treating physician can save a lot of time and effort. If a physician will not release your records to you, ask if he will release them to another one of your physicians. Then, of course, you can ask the second physician for a copy.

Compose your own health history and keep it updated. Be sure to include the name and dosages of current medications, your physician's names and phone numbers, any medication allergies and family contact persons and phone numbers where they can be reached. As many people have coexisting medical problems, it is important that everyone involved with the patient's care have the information. You shouldn't assume that anyone who has an important role in your loved one's care knows his or her entire health history. Repeat it as often as possible and review key points. This is especially critical with physicians and anesthesiologists who are directly responsible for writing patient care orders and managing the patient care.

The U.S. Surgeon General has a Web site that can be used to track your family's health history at https://familyhistory.hhs.gov. (96) This Web site is an easy-to-use format with definitions for the lay person that defines heart disease and many other illnesses. After inputting the family information, it can be saved or printed to bring to your next doctor appointment. As I mentioned earlier, Zebra Health has a health history form that can be downloaded from their Web site. Check Resources Information in the back of this book for the Web site address.

Ask questions and get answers. Keep asking the questions until you get a satisfactory answer. Much of the "hands on" care in the hospital is provided by nurse's aides or Patient Care Technicians, sometimes referred to as Certified Nursing Assistants. Nurse's aides are certified under state regulated programs. There will always be a licensed nurse assigned to your care - either a Licensed Practical Nurse (LPN) or a Registered Nurse (RN). So if someone is telling you to do something that doesn't seem right, ask for your licensed nurse to step into the room. If you do not get satisfaction there, you can ask for a Nurse Manager or Nurse Supervisor on duty. If necessary, ask for the physician to come back to see you or at the very least to call you on the phone. Let your physician know that you want to be involved with your care and that you want to understand the dynamics and factors affecting your care. Sometimes you may need to speak to the doctor directly, whether in a home or hospital setting. Don't be afraid to demand that you speak to the doctor yourself if you feel that it is urgent and a mistake has or will occur if you do not speak to him.

If you are actually hospitalized, try to request a private room. This is not always possible, but allows for the most rest and less chance of contracting an infection or other illness from another patient. The incidence of hospital-induced infections is high. Ask that all staff wash their hands before touching you, especially after you have had a surgical procedure and have a wound where bacteria can enter.

Know what has been ordered and when to expect it. Hospitals are busy places and mistakes can occur. Know the medications that are being given to you as well as the strength and times they should be given. Whenever possible, bring a notepad and pen into the hospital with you and note the names and title of who is coming in your room and what tests (including blood work) are being done. If you are informed about what is expected to happen and when, your stress level should decrease. Also, you will be aware when something does not occur when it should.

Know your rights as a patient. No one can do anything to you that you do not want done. If you are uncomfortable with a test, physician or any other aspect of your medical care, you have the right to a second opinion. It is helpful, whenever possible, to seek that opinion from a physician who is not based at the same hospital as the first physician (if, of course, time is not a critical issue.) Many insurance companies will pay for a second medical opinion. Also be aware that teaching hospitals utilize medical residents, a medical student who has completed his/her classroom training and is working within the hospital to gain expertise and experience working with patients. Many residents are the first to see the patient in a teaching hospital and then report their findings to the attending doctor (your physician). Medical and surgical residents work under your physician with constant communication and guidance. Being a "teaching" patient under the care of medical or surgical residents does not add any cost to your hospital bill. Some residents, depending on their chosen area of specialty, actually perform surgery under the guidance of the attending physician. You have the right to request "no residents" for any or all of or your care when you are in the hospital if you have private medical insurance. However, if your case is complicated, you will have the benefit of seeing several residents who will put their new skills and knowledge together to come up with a diagnosis. You may want to question if medical testing is really necessary, as many new residents like to order the latest medical tests when trying to determine a diagnosis. It is also important to ask the doctor who enters your room about their specialty and credentials. You will be billed for every specialist who comes into your hospital room.

If you are at the hospital for surgery, make sure everyone is clear what part of the body is to be operated on. Some physicians will have you mark your body with a marker pen to avoid confusion. Operating on the wrong body part or wrong side of the body happens more often than anyone would like to admit.

Draw up a living will. This document puts into writing what medical measures you would like or wouldn't want to be taken in the event of a terminal condition or when you are too ill to make decisions for yourself. Encourage loved ones to do the same. An attorney can easily do this. Be sure to have it notarized and have at least two copies. Be sure to list a reliable person who can take responsibility and make medical decisions on your behalf if you are unable to do so. Be sure you have clearly discussed your long-term care with this person and they are agreeable and have it in writing. Whether your patient advocate is a relative or non-relative, you must have a signed, notarized paper authorizing permission for your case to be discussed and/or medical decisions to be made by your advocate on your behalf. Bring notarized copies of your living will to the hospital if the situation warrants it. Although I have these for myself, my advocate has easy access to them and I do not bring them to the hospital at each visit.

In 2002, the Joint Commission and Centers for Medicare and Medicaid launched a "Speak Up" campaign. They encouraged patients to voice their concerns and ask questions. It helps to be polite and friendly. Although you may not be feeling your best, no one will want to deal with you if you are consistently disrespectful or verbally abusive to them. The Speak Up initiative promotes the following:

Speak up if you have questions or concerns; and if you don't understand, ask again. It's your body and you have a right to know.

*P*ay attention to the care you are receiving. Make sure you're getting the right treatments and medications by the right healthcare professionals. Don't assume anything.

*E*ducate yourself about your diagnosis, the medical tests that you are undergoing and your treatment plan.

*A*sk a trusted family member or friend to be your advocate.

*K*now what medication you take and why you take it. Medication errors are the most common healthcare mistake.

*U*se a hospital clinic, surgery center or other type of healthcare organization that has undergone a rigorous on-site evaluation against established state-of-the-art quality and safety standards, such as that provided by the Joint Commission.

*P*articipate in all decisions about your treatment. You are the center of the healthcare team. (97).

The Joint Commission, (JCAHO), the organization responsible for inspections and accreditation of our hospitals and nursing facilities, has various brochures available on their Web site at www.jointcommission.org. The literature that the Joint Commission distributes has actual questions to ask of your healthcare providers to insure that you get the best, safest care.

Many hospitals now use "hospitalists," their own in-hospital staff of doctors, to care for the patient during their stay. These doctors do not personally know the patient or their medical history. They rely on the patient's own internist or sometimes the patient themselves to supply the history. However, a patient in pain or overwhelmed with illness may not be a good historian. It is vital to have another person present at all times possible to supply the information and to listen to the information received. A person under stress simply cannot retain all the information presented or understand it, for that matter. Even the questionnaire forms in the physician offices contain medical words or phrases that the layperson would not be familiar with. An example is the term "SOB" (commonly used as an abbreviation for Shortness of Breath) used on a cardiologist or pulmonary questionnaire. My family member was not familiar with this term and several others on a health questionnaire, although she did experience SOB. It is important that you ask what a word or term means when completing questionnaires if you are not familiar with them.

Although we have made tremendous advances in medical care over the past years, many times it still comes down to the delivery of the care that has the most effect on the patient. I truly believe that hospital administrators, health insurance companies and pharmaceutical companies have lost focus of the patient and have turned their priority to making profits. In turn, the lack of staff, adequate training and time constraints, greatly impacts our healthcare. We have lost touch with the personal, individual care of the patient. As nurses and doctors are rushed to provide care, they sometimes forget to show the kindness, compassion, and empathy that can sometimes do more for healing that a prescription.

Insurance companies mandate earlier discharges from the hospital, sending patients home with little knowledge or little resources to care for themselves. If the physicians and nurses don't have time to educate the patient, the patient will have to educate himself.

Chapter 29

TAKE CONTROL OF YOUR HEALTH

"The road to medical knowledge is through the pathological museum and not through an apothecary's shop." -   William Withey Gull

Taking control of your health means you have to take an active role in your health and your healthcare. You need to educate yourself about your illness, medication, treatments and testing. You need to be proactive and responsible in respect to how you eat, exercise and heed changes in your body.

Ask for a copy of your test results and ask what the implications are. There is less likelihood that something will go unaddressed or missed if you are discussing it together with your physician.   Physicians' offices are busy places, staffed with many people who are responsible for receiving laboratory and other testing results. Sometimes, they get misfiled or misplaced without your physician ever seeing them. Sometimes, the physician just simply forgets to follow up. YOU are responsible for your health. If you have not heard back from a physician regarding a medical test, call his office and ask for the results, preferably in writing. Then educate yourself. Ask questions of your physician or his nurse so that you can better understand your illness, the treatment and expectations. Ask for written material relating to your illness or injury. Most physicians have it readily available and are pleased to give it to you. Some offer informational or preoperative teaching online. I have never had a physician's office charge me for copies of my records. I also make copies of the records that I am given and distribute copies to my other specialists at my next appointment. This allows me the time to verify that this physician is aware of any new findings and provide input to the relevance of my care.

Some physician offices have videos available for their patients to view for educational purposes. Realize that not all will experience the same illness or injury in the same manner. You are an individual so expect that you may experience some and not all of the symptoms of a particular illness or injury.

When recovery from your illness or injury does not progress as you were told it would, call and schedule a follow-up appointment. Don't be afraid to ask your doctor if you should schedule and appointment with a specialist if you are not improving. Most physicians are not threatened by this, and would rather have the input of a physician who specializes in a particular area of medicine.

Educate yourself about your particular illness or health issue. There are reliable consumer health guides available to the public at bookstores and libraries.

Several books that I found to be extremely well written and informational include:

American Medical Association - Complete Home Medical Guide, John Wiley and Sons, Inc. 4th Edition, 2004.
ISBN # 0-471 26911-5

Mayo Clinic Family Health Book - 3rd Edition, Scott C. Litin M.D., Editor in Chief, Harper Resource, Collins, 2003.
ISBN # 0-06 000250-06

John Hopkins Family Health Book, Harpers Collins Publishers, Michael J. Klag, M.D., M. P. H., Editor in Chief, 1999.
ISBN# 0-06 270149-5

In adulthood, there are some important factors that can affect your health. They are your family history, your weight, your emotional state, your overall health and how you address your medical and dental care, destructive vices such as smoking and drinking, underuse or misuse of prescription drugs and the natural aging processes.

Some of these you simply have no control over, such as your family history and natural aging. However, you should be informed about the health history of your parents, siblings and grandparents and share this information with your physician. With this information it is possible to detect or delay damage before it occurs. Early intervention with someone with a family history of diabetes or heart disease can add years to his or her life. Sit down with family members and write out the health issues that affected generations past and present. Share this information with your physician. It may help if you do not identify family members by name, but rather by generation and gender to maintain privacy. Be sure to share your family health history with your relatives, especially when there is the potential for a common illness within the family tree.

Be honest with your physician about your emotional state. It is possible that he/she may be able to help you with medication or suggest someone who can help you. Long-term depression can lead to weight gain, high blood pressure and other related medical illnesses.

Being proactive involves yearly routine medical physicals when you are not ill. A yearly physical allows for a more comprehensive exam by your physician when you are not under duress. He/she can assess all systems of your body during this time.

Physicians typically schedule more time for a well physical exam than for ill visits. This is a good time for your physician to assess your need for vaccine boosters and recommend health-screening examinations that are relevant to your age and health history.

Routine dental checkups are also important. In recent years, gum disease or periodontal disease have been linked to heart attacks and heart infections.

Be honest with your physician regarding the medications that you are or are not taking. If a physician orders a medication and you decide to stop taking it after two days due to side effects, it is important to let him know. Obviously, you may not achieve the full desired effects if you stop taking it early. Antibiotics should always be taken until the prescription runs out unless you are having an adverse effect from them, in which case you need to contact your physician immediately. You most likely will have a relief of your symptoms after 24 hours of antibiotics but it will not be enough to fully eradicate the infection within you. It is very likely that you will redevelop a full-blown infection, which may become resistant to the very antibiotic that was prescribed for you initially.

There has been an increase in the use of naturopathic vitamins and treatments in the past ten years. If you are taking nonprescription medications, including vitamins, it is important to tell your physician. Some of these drugs or vitamins may interact negatively with the ones that your physician prescribes and some may have serious side effects when taken together.

When you are prescribed a new medication, always ask your physician and pharmacist if you can drink alcoholic beverages with the new medication. You should be honest with your physician regarding your daily or weekly intake of alcoholic beverages. Some of your symptoms may be caused by alcohol consumption or abuse and your physician needs to know if this is a factor in your care.

The natural aging process is inevitable. However, we can help ourselves by maintaining proper nutrition and weight. Being overweight has been linked to diabetes and heart disease. Being overweight can also predispose you to sleep apnea that can further stress your heart and cause undue fatigue. Another health issue related to aging is peripheral artery disease. This condition is when the arteries in the legs get blocked or narrowed by plaque. A frequent early sign is aching or burning pain in the legs after walking.

Some medical conditions may be genetically inherited or develop after years of high blood pressure, high cholesterol or diabetes. Early intervention is a must. My own mother ignored her peripheral artery disease symptoms for years and unfortunately had to have her leg amputated. She knew she had waited too long to seek treatment. Usually a venous bypass surgery can be performed early on, which is similar to the technique utilized in a heart bypass.

Healthy veins are used from another part of the body and put in the leg to "get around" the blocked arteries to establish better circulation. There are new treatments being used with balloon angioplasty and thermal ablation to treat peripheral artery disease. These treatments are less invasive than a venous bypass and there is hope on the horizon for those affected by this.

Proper diet and exercise along with early intervention of any existing conditions or health issues related to family history can all help delay premature aging.

Some information that you should know about yourself are: your total cholesterol, your LDL or "bad" cholesterol, your HDL or "good" cholesterol, your triglycerides, your blood pressure and your fasting blood sugar. Your physician can order these blood tests, with the exception of blood pressure, as part of your yearly physical exam. Your blood pressure should be checked at each physician office visit, whether you are ill or not.

Ask your physician what the current range is for your healthy weight. Make every effort to maintain a weight within this range. Calculate your BMI (Body Mass Index) and see where yours falls in relation to what is considered "normal."

Other tests less commonly ordered might also provide useful information for your physician to know about your health. These include a blood test for C-reactive protein, vitamin D level, H. Pylori test and glucose tolerance test.

C-Reactive Protein is a blood test that can indicate inflammation in the body. Although it is not specific to where the inflammation is, it is an indicator that further testing may need to be done. It is believed that an elevated C-reactive protein may indicate impending cardiac trouble, such as heart attack and stroke, among many other illnesses.

Vitamin D is added to the milk we drink. We also get a certain amount of it from the sun. However, newer studies are linking deficiency of vitamin D to cancer. A simple blood test can provide the answer. A deficiency can easily be corrected with vitamin D supplements. Be sure to have your physician monitor your intake if you require supplements, as vitamin D is a fat-soluble vitamin. Fat-soluble vitamins are stored in the liver and excess can cause side effects.

Helicobacter Pylori, otherwise known as H. Pylori, is a bacteria that is associated with stomach ulcers and several other ailments. The prevalence of Helicobacter Pylori infection worldwide is approximately 50%, as high as 80%–90% in developing countries and approximately 35%–40% in the United States. Approximately 20% of persons infected with H. Pylori develop related gastroduodenal disorders during their lifetime. (98) Many of those infected never have outward symptoms. Various methods are used to detect this bacteria, including blood test, stool test, breath test, or the most accurate, a biopsy of the stomach lining taken during an endoscopy. An endoscopy is a procedure where a lighted scope is passed into the stomach by a gastroenterologist. H. Pylori can be treated with antibiotics. The presence of H. Pylori can lead to stomach ulcers, gastritis or possibly promote the growth of cancer over time. Check with your physician regarding testing.

The glucose tolerance test is a good indication of glucose intolerance or diabetes. A blood sample is taken after a period of fasting to determine the blood sugar or glucose level. The patient is then given a bottle of a glucose drink and another blood sample is drawn at 2 hours after the drink. Physicians can see the response of the individual to a predetermined amount of glucose and, based on the results, can determine if a patient is currently a diabetic or is likely to develop diabetes in the future. Some physicians now routinely monitor the blood for A1c (glycosylated hemoglobin) level, which reflects the overall blood glucose levels over the past three months.

Check with your doctor to ensure that your vaccines are up to date. Vaccines are weakened particles of various disease causing germs. There are many vaccines on the market that were not available 50 years ago. Some of these include Hepatitis A & B, HIB, Pneumococcal, Shingles vaccine, HPV for cervical cancer and Zostavax for chicken pox. This is especially important if you are to be traveling in the near future. Many baby boomers received vaccines as young children and may need a "booster" to increase their immunity in later years. If you are injured while traveling and require a tetanus booster, your vaccination may not be covered by your health insurance in a foreign country. It is common sense to keep your vaccinations up to date.

The Centers for Disease Control maintains a Web site at www.cdc.gov, which details the need for vaccines and immunizations and the recommended intervals. These vaccines are not always without risk, so be sure to discuss them with your physician prior to injection. Sometimes vaccines can cause serious side effects. Generally the benefits outweigh the risks.

Millions of people get vaccines yearly with no ill side effects. By the age of 6 years, children in the United States will have received about 10 routine immunizations, which are administered in approximately 30 injections. Some children are given up to 5 different vaccines in one office visit. More recently, Thimerosal an additive to multi-use vaccine vials has come under scrutiny. It has been used as a preservative in many drug products since the 1930's. Thimerosal has been suspected as a cause for mercury toxicity and possibly autism. Most single-dose vials of vaccines do not contain Thimerosal. This is usually not as cost effective for your physician, but you can ask him to order it as a single dose from your pharmacy. You may also experience difficulty with insurance coverage if you decide to seek this route. The benefits of vaccines have helped us to virtually eradicate many diseases that were prevalent 50 years ago.

Vaccines are necessary under law prior to admission into school. Some waivers are allowed in the case of religious objection.

Flu vaccines have also been known to save lives, especially among the elderly and immuno-compromised patients. The flu vaccine also has its limitations. In order to have enough of a vaccine available for the fall and winter months, scientists have to develop a vaccine based on the various strains of influenza that are anticipated for the upcoming season. The vaccine may not be effective with the current strain of flu that is circulating. According to the Centers for Disease Control, the 2007-2008 flu vaccine was only about 44% effective. Be sure to check with your physician to see if he advises that you should receive it. Many communities hold flu inoculation clinics at low cost. Check with your local public health department for resources near you.

Newer vaccines come on the market every few years. One of the newer ones is Gardasil. You will need to discuss with your physician if this vaccine against the Human Papilloma Virus is appropriate for yourself (females only) or daughter(s). My under-standing is that currently it only protects against four types of HPV, of which there are many. Since 2006, is it estimated that 1 in 4 young women have received the Gardasil vaccine.

Chapter 30

FIGHTING FOR YOUR LIFE - REJECTED CLAIMS

"Extreme remedies are very appropriate for extreme diseases." - Hippocrates

Even though you may have a wonderful health insurance plan, at some point, you may be at odds with your health care provider in regard to coverage. The last 20 years has been a revolving door regarding health care insurance coverage and pre-authorization for testing and/or surgery. The private health insurance companies took a more active role in deciding who would be covered under their policy for an array of services. This struggle for control of your health care continues today. Some have accused the health care insurance industry of trying to practice medicine without a license. If your physician orders an expensive test or procedure and your insurance company decides that they will not pay, what is the patient to do?

One of the most recent issues to come under scrutiny is the concern of overuse of advanced medical scans, such as CAT scans, PET scans and even MRIs. Medical insurance companies cite concerns regarding excess radiation exposure in addition to the high cost of the testing. In the year 2000, on average there were 12 scans performed per 100 people. In the year 2005 that figure nearly doubled to 22 scans per 100 people. (99) With private health insurers and governmental programs, such as Medicare, reimbursing less for medical expenses, facilities that have their own scanners stand to make a substantial profit from ordering a large volume of scans. The makers of the scanning machines market them aggressively. Consideration to require pre-authorization from an insurance provider for more routine testing such as EKG's and echocardiograms was attempted in New Jersey but recently stopped. (100) Physician groups argue with health insurance carriers regarding these issues frequently necessitating physician offices and hospitals to hire personnel to act as a liaison with medical insurance carriers to substantiate claims for medical testing. Coverage for procedures and testing will continue to be an issue as health insurance providers strive to place limitations on their covered expenses.

Before agreeing to an expensive medical test such as a CAT scan or MRI, ask your physician a few questions.

- Why is this test necessary?

- Are there other test options?

- Is there any risk associated with this test?

- Will this test give you insight regarding my treatment from here on forward?

- How certain are you about my diagnosis before I have this test?

- Can I safely wait a period of time before having this test done?

Some physicians will order expensive testing due to the limited time they now have to evaluate a patient in the office. An MRI, PET scan or Cat scan can offer quick answers as to whether there is something growing where it shouldn't be, allay patient fears and provide some protection against malpractice claims (assuming the test is interpreted correctly!) Radioactive isotopes are injected into your vein to enhance the views during some MRI's, Pet scans and Cat scans. Although the risks are small, there are some that may experience an allergic reaction to these chemicals or even permanent damage to the kidneys. It is important to answer all pre-test questions honestly at the time of your examination and follow post-test instructions carefully. Be sure to request a copy of a written report and a copy of the test on CD-ROM on the day of the examination. A CD can usually be made within minutes after the completion of the testing. If you move, go to another hospital or change physicians, a copy of your exam on CD or a written copy may save you from having the test repeated.

As with everything else I have come up against, I have determined that it is in your best interest to put up a valiant fight for your rights. This may be especially true for new drug treatments, new tests and new medical procedures. It wasn't that many years ago that kidney transplants, liver transplants, heart and lung transplants were all considered experimental and not covered by insurance. As time has progressed, these procedures are considered more of the normal and covered by our healthcare insurers. Not all insurers will feel the same as you or I. Be prepared for the fight of your life but know that it is possible to win with persistence. You may have to devote a lot of time and energy into an appeal but it can be worth it in the end.

Get started immediately. Over time, you may forget the details of your claim, so take the time to jot them down immediately and start the appeal process. Some insurance companies will place a limit on the period of time in which you have to appeal. So start as soon as possible when the information is fresh in your mind.

First, you need to read your policy for coverage, limitations and exclusions. Your employer may have a human resources person responsible for and knowledgeable of the health care coverage policy. Utilize this person as much as possible to better your understanding of the policy and what is covered and what is not.

Be organized and gather all the relevant information. You will need dates and names of people who you speak with regarding this issue, so be sure to start a notebook and date and time each call along with the name of the person you speak with. It can help to have a callback number for the contact person, but many will not give their last name or extension number. You can ask for an "incident" number or unique identifying number that confirms your communication with someone at the company.

Follow up and follow through. Just because someone promises you something over the phone it does not mean it will occur. You may need to ask to speak to a supervisor who usually has more authority in making critical decisions for the company. You can also ask for written confirmation regarding your telephone conversation in the form of a follow-up letter in the mail. It is always best to get the information in writing. Not all phone representatives are created equal. I have been known to hang up and start over again if I come up against a hostile or unsympathetic telephone consultant. Ask your insurance carrier if they have a nurse case manager who you can speak with. Be sure to get a telephone number where you can call the individual back if it is necessary. Get the names, dates and time that you spoke to someone and write them down. Keep all your information together in a file folder.

If a phone call to the insurer does not get a positive outcome, you will need to put your issue in writing. Make sure to include copies of any paperwork, but be sure to keep the originals in a safe location. Whenever possible, enlist your physician to write a letter on your behalf regarding the rejected claim. Ask for a copy of your physician's letter to be sent to you for your records. He/she can add specific information regarding abnormal test results or implications of withholding treatments.

The Kaiser Family Foundation is a nonprofit, private organization that has up-to-date information of all states' health information online at: www.kff.org. On their Web site, you can link to your specific state for current state policies regarding health care.

Don't give up. I usually advise that you can do this appeal process yourself or have a family member assist you. If you need other assistance, you may want to contact a support group associated with similar issues, your state or federal insurance departments, a state legislator or a lawyer, if necessary. It is estimated that close to 50 percent of those who do appeal will win their case. (101)

In 2007, a 17-year-old girl died while her family fought their insurance provider for coverage of a liver transplant. Ironically, the insurance provider reversed their decision and had agreed to cover the cost of the surgery just hours prior to the girl's death. (102) Up to 150 nurses and teens had stood outside CIGNA corporate offices to protest the original decision.

When applying for Social Security disability benefits historically, applicants were denied several times before benefits would be approved retroactively. I personally knew of four such cases. Only one of the four was approved the first time and I am proud to say that it was a relative of mine for whom I filled out the paperwork. Sadly, her death occurred within two months of being accepted for benefits. I understand that no one wants to make it easy for those who may not qualify for benefits, but it just seemed cruel in the other cases that their denials could drag on for close to a year. These women were seriously ill, they could not work and they had no benefits coming in. With good record keeping, patience and persistence, a person can handle their own appeals. However, there are plenty of lawyers and other groups willing to assist a person with Social Security Denial Appeals for a portion of the retroactive benefits.

Medicare can also deny claims, and you should use the same process as above to appeal. See contact information in the Resources Information section at the end of this book.

Organ Transplants

If you are waiting for an organ transplant, you can increase your odds of getting a transplant by getting on several waiting lists. You will want to be close to and choose a transplant center that does a high volume of these surgeries with a high success rate.

This is another example where checking the credentials of both the transplant facility and the surgeon is crucial. The surgeon should be board certified and should be a member of the American Society of Transplant Surgeons. Generally, you want a surgeon who performs a large volume of these surgeries yearly and who has performed hundreds of these transplants in his lifetime.

Each state has its own laws regarding organ donation, and the donor must have made a declaration during their lifetime that they desire to donate an organ or organs. The donor's family does not need to pay for the harvesting surgery nor do they receive any type of payment for donating a family member's organs.

All United States organ donations are governed by The National Organ Transplant Act, Public Law 98-507. Organs cannot be bought or sold in the United States and how much money you have or earn will not allow you to get an organ sooner. All those awaiting a transplant must be placed on a waiting list until a matching organ can be located, unless they are fortunate enough to have a family member directly donate one to them.

Likewise, HMO's are being held more accountable for deaths linked to their refusal to pay for treatments and procedures (such as organ transplants).

Chapter 31

THE BOTTOM LINE

"Every human being is the author of his own health or disease." - Hindu Prince Guatama Siddharta, the founder of Buddhism

When it comes to your health, you are the expert. You need to be responsible for your own health, maintaining a healthy lifestyle, keeping track of your medical history and scheduling an annual physical with your private physician. You can choose to follow your physician's advice or not, but be prepared to suffer the consequences or pay the price if things don't go as you had planned.

Your physician should have a collateral relationship with you based on good communication and thorough examination. He/she should respect your opinions and decisions and you should respect theirs. Your interactions should never be in a condescending or patronizing manner.

If you have a problem that does not resolve after a physician's treatment and you feel that something is still "wrong" don't be afraid to ask your physician some key questions. Ask "Could something else be wrong?" or "If it isn't this, what could it be and how can we find out?" When all else fails, don't be afraid of seeking care somewhere else or obtaining a second opinion. Only you know your body and what you are experiencing. Always trust your instinct.

Do not consent to a procedure or surgery unless a physician or surgeon you trust and respect has answered all your questions and presented any alternative options.

Remember, medicine is not an exact science!

RESOURCES INFORMATION

The Internet has evolved into a wonderful learning and resource tool. Having said that, I don't advise you to use the Internet to solely diagnose or attempt to medically treat yourself or your family. However, with the guidance of your physician, the Internet can be useful in gathering additional information. I highly recommend well-known Web sites that are associated with National Foundations, such as the American Heart Association, American Cancer Society or others. Message boards are also available online and can serve as a support group for people who are suffering from similar illnesses. However, remember that you are an individual and not all treatments will work for everyone. Be sure to discuss any change in treatment with your physician so that your specific needs may be evaluated and not cause additional harm or injury.

I have added a few reputable Web sites and other resources below.

REFERENCE BOOKS:

For excellent medical reference books, check your local library for these titles:

American Medical Association - Complete Home Medical Guide, John Wiley and Sons, Inc. 4th Edition, 2004
ISBN # 0-471 26911-5

Mayo Clinic Family Health Book - 3rd Edition, Scott C. Litin M.D., Editor in Chief, Harper Resource, 2003.
ISBN # 0-06 000250-06

John Hopkins Family Health Book, Harpers Collins Publishers, Michael J. Klag, M.D., M. P. H., Editor in Chief, 1999 – ISBN# 0-06 270149-5(57)

The Physicians Desk Reference, (PDR) has been the physicians' standard for years regarding medications. Most libraries will have a copy in their reference section. Such information can be accessed on the Internet, however, you must subscribe to a full version. This site offers easy-to-read and understandable information regarding medications for the layperson.
Internet address: PDRHealth at www. pdrhealth.com

Worst Pills, Best Pills, A Consumer's Guide to Avoiding Drug-Induced Death or Illness," in collaboration with Larry D. Sasich, Pharm D., M.P.H., and Rose Ellen Hope, R. Ph., Pocket Books, 1999, ISBN # 067101918X

ILLNESS/DISEASE INFORMATION AND SUPPORT:

Medline Plus - this site is from the National Library of Medicine and contains information regarding specific diseases, support groups and articles.
U.S. National Library of Medicine
8600 Rockville Pike
Bethesda, MD 20894
Internet address: www.medlineplus.gov.

NORD - The National Organization for Rare Diseases
Some diseases that are not as common are discussed here. There is a database that can be accessed to learn about rare diseases and investigative treatments and new drug therapies for rare illnesses. This Web site is easy to use, contains helpful information with addresses, phone numbers and support groups.
National Organization for Rare Disorders
55 Kenosia Avenue PO Box 1968
Danbury, CT 06813-1968
Tel: (203) 744-0100 Toll free: (800) 999-6673 (voicemail only)
Fax Number: (203)798-2291
E-mail Contact: orphan@rarediseases.org
Internet address: http://www.rarediseases.org

Health finder - A web site sponsored by the United States Department of Health and Welfare which offers an array of articles not only related to specific illnesses, but health care and safety in general. In addition to a medical dictionary, this Web site also includes information on prevention, medical alternatives and medicine interactions. A truly diverse site.
National Health Information Center
P.O. Box 1133, Washington, DC 20013-1133
Internet address: www.healthfinder.gov.

American Academy of Family Physicians
This site offers a Self-Care section, lists a number of symptoms and suggests when to call your doctor. Some of the highlights are sections related to Healthy Living, Men, Women, a Smart Patient Guide, Advocacy, Over the Counter Guide, Parents and Kids, Seniors Section and Health Tools such as a medical dictionary.
Phone: 800-274-2237
Email: contactcenter@aafp.org
Internet address: www.familydoctor.org

UpToDate, Inc.
95 Sawyer Road
Waltham, MA 02453
Technical medical information regarding many illnesses and diseases.
Be sure to click on the "For patients" tab and perform a search for the desired topic.
Internet address: www.uptodate.com

National Center for Biotechnology Information, part of the U.S. National Institutes of Health
A technical Web site with medical journal articles on many topics.
National Institutes of Health (NIH)
9000 Rockville Pike
Bethesda, Maryland 20892
Internet address: www.pubmed.gov

U. S. Department of Health and Social Services
Agency for Research and Healthcare Quality
U.S. Department of Health & Human Services
200 Independence Avenue
S.W. · Washington, D.C. 20201
This is an informative Web site with many health-related topics.
Internet address: http://www.ahrq.gov/consumer/

CANCER INFORMATION AND SUPPORT:

SHARE - speak to a breast cancer survivor on the phone - a
network of breast and ovarian cancer survivors.
1501 Broadway
Suite 704A
New York, New York 10036
Phone: 212-719-0364
Toll-free: 1-866-891-2392
Fax: 212-869-3431

Breast Cancer Network of Strength -
Breast Cancer Network of Strength Headquarters
212 W. Van Buren, Suite 1000
Chicago, IL 60607-3903
Tel: 312-986-8338
Tel: 1-800-221-2141
Fax: 312-294-8597

Gilda's Club - Free support group for anyone living with cancer
Email: info@gildasclub.org
Write: Gilda's Club Worldwide
322 Eighth Avenue, Suite 1402
New York, NY 10001
Gilda's Club
Phone: 888-GILDA-4-U
www.gildasclub.org

Breast Cancer Action - information for those diagnosed with Breast Cancer
55 New Montgomery Street
Suite 323
San Francisco, CA 94105
Phone: 415.243.9301
877-2STOPBC (877-278-6722) Toll Free
Fax: 415-243-3996
Email: info@bcaction.org
Web site: www.bcaction.org

Susan G. Komen for the Cure - support and information for those diagnosed with Breast Cancer
5005 LBJ Freeway
Suite 250
Dallas, TX 75244
United States
Tel: 877 GO KOMEN (1-877-465-6636)
www.Komen.org

The Susan Love Research Foundation- for those diagnosed with Breast Cancer
2811 Wilshire Blvd., Suite 500
Santa Monica, California 90404
Fax: 310-828-5403
Phone: 310-828-0060 (local) or 1-866-569-0388
Web site: www.susanlovemd.com

Get Breast Cancer Facts
Sponsored by Astra Zeneca Pharmaceuticals
Get Breast Cancer Facts
www.getbcfacts.com
You can contact the Astra Zeneca Cancer Support Network at:
Telephone: 1-866-99-AZCSN

FORCE: Facing Our Risk of Cancer Empowered
16057 Tampa Palms Blvd. W, PMB #373
Tampa, FL 33647
(954) 255-8732
Toll-free voice mail: (866)288-RISK
Fax: (954)827-2200
Email: info@facingourrisk.org
Helpline: 866-824-RISK (7475)

American Cancer Society
(Free or low-cost pap smears and pelvic exams)
Phone Number: 1-800-227-2345
Internet Address: http://www.cancer.org

National Cervical Cancer Coalition (NCCC)
(Free or low-cost pap smears and pelvic exams)
Phone Number: (800) 685-5531
Internet Address: http://www.nccc-online.org/

CancerCare - is a national nonprofit organization that provides free, professional support services to anyone affected by cancer.
www.cancercare.org
1-800-813-HOPE
CancercareCopay.org - for those experiencing difficulties meeting insurance co-pay for prescription medication related to cancer.
1-866-55-COPAY

Cancer.net - information from the American Society of Clinical Oncology
Mailing address: American Society of Clinical Oncology, 2318 Mill Road, Suite 800, Alexandria, VA 22314, Attn: Communications and Patient Information Department
Web Site - www.cancer.net
Email: contactus@cancer.net
Phone: 571-483-1780 or 888-651-3038 Fax: 571-366-9537

Cancer Clinical Trials
1-800-303-5691
www.cancer.org/clinical trials

CHECKING MEDICAL CREDENTIALS INCLUDING BOARD CERTIFICATION:

American Board of Medical Specialties
To check if a physician is board certified or find a board-certified physician
Tel: 866-275-2267
Internet address: www.abms.org

American Society of Plastic Surgeons
Plastic Surgery Educational Foundation
444 E. Algonquin Rd.
Arlington Heights, IL 60005
Tel: 847-228-9900
 Internet address: www.plasticsurgery.org.
You are able to search for an accredited physician by name, location, or zip code.

Federation of State Medical Boards of the United States, Inc.
PO Box 619850
Dallas, TX 75261-9850
Main phone: (817) 868-4000
State Medical Boards (continued)
Main fax: (817) 868-4099
Internet address: http://www.fsmb.org/
Click on the State Medical Board Directory.
Offers instant access to a database containing reprimand board actions taken against physicians. A small fee is necessary to access this information and must be paid for with a credit card.
Internet address: www.docinfo.org.
Internet address: www.fsmb.org - Click on State Medical Board Directory

Each state also has a Medical Board. Be sure to check your specific State Board regarding your physician's current licensure or infractions. Check with your State Department of Health.

American College of Surgeons
Members of the American College of Surgeons as well as information regarding second opinions, information about undergoing surgery and other helpful information.
American College of Surgeons
633 N. Saint Clair Street
Chicago, Ill. 60611-3211
Tel: 312-202-5000
Toll Free 1-800-621-4111
Fax 312-202-5001
E-mail: postmaster@facs.org
Internet address: www.facs.org

American Medical Association
515 N. State Street
Chicago, IL 60610
(800) 621-8335
You can research your physician's medical training and whether or not she/he is board certified in a specific specialty. Some also have office locations and phone numbers.
 The American Board of Medical Specialties can verify whether a doctor is board certified at www.abms.org/newsearch.asp.
Internet address: www.ama-assn.org

American College of Physicians
Information regarding physician members.
American College of Physicians
190 North Independence Mall West
Philadelphia, PA 19106-1572
Toll Free: (800)-523-1546
 Local: (215)-351-2400
Internet address: www.acponline.org

Health Grades - This site allows you to research physicians, hospitals and nursing homes. Be advised that you must pay for reports and log in to the site.
Health Grades, Inc.
500 Golden Ridge Road, Suite 100
Golden, CO 80401
(303) 716-0041
Internet address: - www.healthgrades.com.

Castle Connolly Medical Ltd. - Assistance in finding a "Top Doctor" or hospital.
42 West 24th Street, 2nd Floor
New York, NY 10010
Tel. (212) 367-8400
Fax (212) 367-0964
Internet address: www.castleconnolly.com.

New York Magazine - to find physicians in the tri-state area of New York, New Jersey, and Connecticut.
New York Media
75 Varick Street
New York, NY, 10013
New York Magazine (continued)
212-508-0700
Top Docs List
Internet address: http://nymag.com/bestdoctors/

Connecticut Magazine - to find physicians in Connecticut who other physicians have recommended.
Connecticut Magazine Staff Directory
Business and Editorial Offices
35 Nutmeg Drive, Trumbull, CT 06611
(203) 380-6600
Business Fax: (203) 380-6610
Editorial Fax: (203) 380-6612
Top Docs List: www.connecticutmag.com

RateMD's - use this site to either rate your MD or check ratings on physicians - by patients for patients
Internet address: www.Ratemds.com

Vitals.com - provides consumers with background information on physicians such as schools attended, board certification, publication and malpractice. Also has a section for consumers to rate a physician.
Internet address: www.Vitals.com

American Massage Therapy Association
Massage Therapist Practice Laws - regulated by each state
Search "states" - to check your state regulation
Internet Web site: www.amtamassage.org

WHERE TO CHECK FACILITY CREDENTIALS:

To check on a hospital:
The Joint Commission on Accreditation of Healthcare Organizations
A nonprofit organization that is responsible for accrediting and certifying hospitals, freestanding surgical centers, physician offices, nursing homes and other health care related institutions in the United States to verify that they meet specific standards. You can also view any special awards given to an institution.
The Joint Commission
One Renaissance Blvd.
Oakbrook Terrace, IL 60181
Tel:(630) 792-5000
Internet address: www.jcaho.org and look under Quality Check.
JACHO Complaints:
Complaints about a health care organization
Tel:800-994-6610
Email: complaint@jointcommission.org

U. S. News and World Report
Corporate Offices
450 W. 33rd Street, 11th Floor
New York, NY 10001
212-716-6800
If you want to find the "best" teaching hospitals according to U.S. News and World Report
Internet address:
www.usnews.com/usnews/nycu/health/hosptl/tophosp.htm.

U.S. Department of Health & Human Services
200 Independence Avenue, S.W.
Washington, D.C. 20201
Review and compare nursing homes and access inspection reports.
Internet address: www.medicare.gov

Joint Commission on Accreditation of Healthcare Organizations
To check hospital accreditation by JACHO
The Joint Commission
One Renaissance Blvd.
Oakbrook Terrace, IL 60181
Internet address: www.qualitycheck.org.
Simply submit your zip code, the hospital zip code or name of the hospital you wish to check.

The Leap Frog Group
Rating of units including high-risk medical procedures.
The Leapfrog Group
c/o Academy Health
1150 17th Street NW, Suite 600
Washington DC 20036
Telephone: 202-292-6713
Fax: 202-292-6813
Email: info@leapfroggroup.org
Internet address: www.leapfroggroup.org

U.S. Department of Health and Human Services
Compare hospitals within your local area. Select three hospitals at a
time to compare side-by-side. Includes patient survey responses to
in-patient care and environment.
U.S. Department of Health & Human Services
200 Independence Avenue, S. W.
Washington, D.C. 20201
Internet address: www.hospitalcompare.hhs.gov

WHERE TO REGISTER A COMPLAINT AGAINST A HEALTHCARE FACILITY:

Joint Commission on Accreditation of Healthcare Organizations
The Joint Commission Complaint Line
One Renaissance Blvd.
Oakbrook Terrace, IL 60181
All complaints are kept confidential.
Complaint Line -1 800-994-6610
Email: complaint@jcaho.org
Internet address: http://www.jointcommission.org/
Internet address: complaint@jcaho.org

YOUR MEDICAL RIGHTS:

HIPAA Rights
U.S. Department of Health & Human Services
200 Independence Avenue, S.W.
Washington, D.C. 20201
Complaints:
Tel: 1-800-368-1019
Internet address: www.hhs.gov/ocr/hipaa

Medicare Rights
520 Eighth Ave.
North Wing, 3rd Fl.
New York, NY 10018
Tel: 212-869-3850 1-888-466-9050
Fax: 212-869-3532
Medicare Appeals
Internet address: www.medicarerights.org

Consumer Bill of Rights
U.S. Office of Personnel Management
1900 E Street NW
 Washington, DC 20415
Tel: (202) 606-1800 | TTY (202) 606-2532
 Internet address: http://www.opm.gov/insure/health/billrights.asp

OMBUDSMAN/PATIENT ADVOCATES/HOSPITAL BILLING
ERRORS:

The National Long Term Care Ombudsman Resource Center - For
State by State listing of Ombudsman
ORC OFFICE
1828 L Street, NW
Suite 801
Washington, DC 20036
Phone - 202-332-2275
The National Long Term Care Ombudsman Resource (continued)
Internet address:
http://www.ltcombudsman.org/static_pages/ombudsmen_list.cfm

Patient Advocates
Helps attain access to care and preserve financial stability related to
disease or illness.
Patient Advocate Foundation
700 Thimble Shoals Blvd.
Suite 200

Patient Advocates – (continued)
Newport News, VA 23606
Phone:1 (800) 532-5274
Fax:(757) 873-8999
Email: info@patientadvocate.org
Internet address: http://www.patientadvocate.org/

Medical Billing Advocates of America
MBAA Corporate Headquarters
Pat Palmer, President
PO Box 1705
Salem, VA 24153
Email: Pat@billadvocates.com
For assistance with Hospital/ Medical Billing issues, contact:
www.billadvocates.com
Phone – 540-387-5870

PHARMACEUTICAL CLINICAL TRIALS - RESEARCH AND
STUDY PROGRAMS:

To find a clinical research study:
If you, a family member or friend is not responding to conventional
treatment, you may want to consider joining a research study. Be
sure to ask your physician about this and he/she may be best able to
guide you to one. However, you can find government-sponsored
studies through the United States National Institute of Health.
National Institutes of Health
9000 Rockville Pike
Bethesda, Maryland 20892
Tel: 301-496-4000,
TTY 301-402-9612
Email: NIHinfo@od.nih.gov
Internet address: www.clinicaltrials.gov.

To locate pharmaceutical industry-sponsored studies at the FDA
U.S. Food and Drug Administration ·
5600 Fishers Lane
Rockville, MD 20857-0001 ·
Tel: 1-888-INFO-FDA (1-888-463-6332)
CenterWatch.com
Internet address: www.centerwatch.com.

Clinical Trials:
Center for Information and Study on Clinical Research Participation
Internet address: www.CISCRP.org

Brochure for those considering clinical trials:
Internet address: www.cdcnpin.org/Brochures/ResStudy.pdf

PRESCRIPTION MEDICATION INFORMATION:

The Physicians Desk Reference (PDR) has been the physicians'
standard for years regarding medications.   Now, such information
can be accessed on the Internet, however, you must subscribe to a
full version.
This site offers easy-to-read and understandable information
regarding medications for the layperson.
Internet address: PDRHealth at www. pdrhealth.com

Medline Plus
U.S. National Library of Medicine - National Institutes of Health
8600 Rockville Pike
Bethesda, MD 20894
The format is easy to read and understand. This site provides
information regarding the use of a drug, the side effects and cautions
related to its use.
Internet address:
http://www.nlm.nih.gov/medlineplus/druginformation.html

FREE AND LOW COST MAMMOGRAMS/PAP SMEARS:

Free Mammograms
American Cancer Society - 1-800-ACS-2345
National Cancer Institute - 1-800-4-CANCER
American Breast Cancer Foundation
Internet address: www.ABCF.org

Free Pap Smears
Pap tests by contacting the National Women's Health Information
Center (NWHIC) at 1-800-994-9662 or the following organizations:
Cancer Information Service, NCI, NIH, HHS
Phone Number: (800) 422-6237
Internet Address: http://cis.nci.nih.gov/

Planned Parenthood Federation of America
(Free or low-cost pap smears and pelvic exams)
Phone Number: (800) 230-7526
Internet Address: http://www.ppfa.org

Free Mammograms and Pap Smears - for those with low income/no
insurance:
National Breast and Cervical Cancer Early Detection Program.
Centers for Disease Control and Prevention
Division of Cancer Prevention and Control
4770 Buford Hwy, NE
MS K-64
Atlanta, GA 30341-3717
Tel: 1 (800) CDC-INFO - 1-888-643-2584
TTY: 1 (888) 232-6348
FAX: (770) 488-4760
E-mail: cdcinfo@cdc.gov

FREE SCREENINGS

Vascular Disease
Sponsored by the Society of Interventional Radiology
Usually held in September
www.legsforlife.org

Depression
Sponsored by Mental Health, Inc.
Usually in October
www.mentalhealthscreening.org

Memory-Alzheimer's
Alzheimer's Foundation of America
Usually in November
www.nationalmemoryscreening.org

Heart Disease
Offered by Sister to Sister (in 19 states)
Offers cholesterol and blood pressure screening
Usually held in February
www.sistertosister.org

Skin Cancer
Sponsored by the American Academy of Dermatology
Usually offered in May
www.aad.org

Asthma
Screening offered by the American College of Allergy, Asthma and
Immunology
250 sites, usually in May
www.acaai.org (click on Pt. education)

FINANCIAL ASSISTANCE:

Department of Health and Human Services
U.S. Department of Health & Human Services
200 Independence Avenue, S.W.
Washington, D.C. 20201
Click on "Find Help, Health Care regardless of you ability to pay."
Internet address: www.hrsa.gov
Patient Assistance Programs - for medications

Bureau of Primary Health. The Department of Health and Human Services.
Federally funded health primary care facilities across the nation for at-risk communities and for those with no health insurance.
A list of facilities can be accessed by state on their Web site.
U.S. Department of Health & Human Services
200 Independence Avenue S.W.
Washington, D.C. 20201
Internet address: http://ask.hrsa.gov/pc/

Insure Kids Now
U.S. Department of Health & Human Services
200 Independence Avenue
S.W. · Washington, D.C. 20201
Tel: 1-877-KIDS-NOW
www.insurekidsnow.net

Needy Meds, Inc
P.O. Box 219
Gloucester, MA 01931
Needy Meds, Inc.
FAX: 1-419-858-7221
*Note this company does not provide telephone assistance. Those needing assistance should refer to the Internet address.
Internet address: www.needymeds.com

RX Assist
Volunteers in Health Care
111 Brewster Street
Pawtucket, RI 02860
Phone: 401-729-3284
Fax: 401-729-2955
Email: info@rxassist.org
Internet address: www.rxassist.com

Medication Discount Cards
Medicare - 1-800-Medicare
Together RX Access 1-800-444-4106
Internet address: http://www.togetherrxaccess.com/Tx/jsp/home.jsp
Pharmaceutical Companies
Johnson and Johnson 1-888-4PP-ANOW
Pfizer 1-866-776-3700
Pfizer - 1-866-706-2400 - for uninsured or underinsured persons
requiring prescription Pfizer brand medications.
www.pfizerhelpfulanswers.com

Assistance with pharmacy costs
Internet address: Togetherrxaccess.com

The Kaiser Family Foundation
Headquarters
2400 Sand Hill Road
Menlo Park, CA 94025
Tel: (650) 854-9400
Fax: (650) 854-4800
Internet address: www.kff.org

ELECTRONIC SECOND OPINION:

Electronic Second Opinion:
Cleveland Clinic
Cleveland Clinic and Partner's Center for Connected Health.

Electronic Second Opinion (continued)
Tel: 800.223.2273
Email: Webmail@ccf.org
Internet address: http://www.eclevelandclinic.org/eCCHome.jsp

DEFECTIVE PHARMACEUTICALS OR MEDICAL DEVICES:

United States Food and Drug Administration
U.S. Food and Drug Administration
5600 Fishers Lane
Rockville, MD 20857-0001
1-888-INFO-FDA (1-888-463-6332)
To read reports online of various medications
Report adverse pharmaceutical or medical device reactions - reporting available online.
Internet address: www.fda.com

FDA MedWatch
FDA - list of recalled or contaminated medications
Internet address: www.fda.gov.medwatch/index.html
Sign up for automatic e-mail alerts:
Internet address:
https://www.accessdata.fda.gov/scripts/medwatch/medwatch-online.htm

WHERE TO CREATE YOUR OWN FAMILY HEALTH HISTORY ONLINE:

U. S. Surgeon General has a Web site that can be used to track your family's health history
U.S. Department of Health & Human Services
200 Independence Avenue S.W.
Washington, D.C. 20201
Internet address: https://familyhistory.hhs.gov/

326

Zebra Health
Download a Personal Health Record
Internet address: www.zebrahealth.com

PERSONAL MEDICATION RECORD

AARP: www.aarp.org/health/rx_drugs/usingmeds
Print out a personal medication record

FOREIGN TRAVEL INFORMATION AND GUIDELINES:

Bureau of Consular Affairs - U. S. Department of State
Office of Overseas Citizen Service - within State Department
Bureau of Consular Affairs
Emergency number: 1-888-407-4747
In the U.S. or Canada - 202-501-4444
Internet address:
http://travel.state.gov/travel/tips/brochures/brochures_1215.html.

Center for Disease Control (CDC) Atlanta, Georgia - pertaining to travel in foreign countries
Centers for Disease Control and Prevention
1600 Clifton Rd, Atlanta, GA 30333, U.S.A.
Public Inquiries: (404) 498-1515 / (800) 311-3435
International Traveler's Hotline - 1-877-FYI -TRIP (1-877-394-8747)
FAX 1-888-CDC FAXX (1-888-232-3299)
Internet address: www.cdc.gov/travel

Joint Commission International - to check accredited medical facilities outside of the United States
The Joint Commission
One Renaissance Blvd.
Oakbrook Terrace, IL 60181
Internet address: www.jointcommissioninternational.org
Tel: 630-792-5800

U. S. State Department
Bureau of Public Affairs
Public Communication Division
PA/PL, Room 2206
U.S. Department of State
Washington, DC 20520
Tel: (202) 647-6575
Email through: http://contact-us.state.gov/
Register your travel plans with the State Department through a free online service.
Internet address: https://travelregistration.state.gov.

A Web site that lists names of companies that can provide health insurance in foreign countries as well as air evacuation during a medical emergency.
InsureMyTrip.com
World Headquarters
100 Commerce Drive
Warwick, Rhode Island
02886 USA
Customer Service:
Telephone: 1-800- 487-4722
401-773-9300
Fax: 401-921-4530
Internet address: www.Insuremytrip.com

International Association for Medical Assistance to Travelers - This Web site can recommend English-speaking doctors in foreign countries.
Internet address: www.iamat.org

Access-Able Travel Source
Information about traveling with disabilities and handicapped access to cruise ships, hotels and cities.
www.access-able.com

World Health Organization
Current illness and health threats around the world on this site.
Internet address: www.who.int

HEALTH SAVINGS PLAN INFORMATION:

Information on Flexible Health Savings Plans
U. S. Department of Bureau of Labor Statistics
U.S. Bureau of Labor Statistics
Postal Square Building
2 Massachusetts Avenue N.E.
Washington, DC 20212-0001
Tel: (202) 691-5200
Internet address: www.bls.gov

USED MEDICATION DISPOSAL:

The Star Fish Project - to donate used medication
Center for Special Studies
New York-Presbyterian Hospital
Weill Cornell Medical Center
119 West 24 Street
New York, NY 10011
Tel: (212) 746-7164
Fax: (212) 746-8415
Email: info@thestarfishproject.org
Internet address: www.thestarfishproject.org

Prescription Drug Repository - Missouri
Medical Missions for Christ Community Health Center
1193 Highway KK, Suite B
P.O. Box 1327
Osage Beach, Missouri 65065
Tel: 573-348-9444
Internet address:
http://www.dhss.mo.gov/DrugRepository/FAQs.html

Oklahoma Drug donations:
Oklahoma Board of Pharmacy
4545 Lincoln Blvd., Ste 112
Oklahoma City, OK 73105
Tel: 405-521-3815
Fax: 405-521-3758
Internet address: pharmacy@pharmacy.ok.gov
Internet address:
http://www.ok.gov/OSBP/documents/unused%2007-05.pdf

COMPLEMENTARY AND ALTERNATIVE MEDICINE:

National Center for Complementary and Alternative Medicine - sponsored by the U.S. National Institutes of Health
Internet address: www.naccam.nih.gov

Lotus Medical - An educational Web site to promote healing and health by exploring various healing traditions including herbal treatments, Pilates and colonics. Located in the northeastern United States with monthly meetings held. Open to health care professionals.
http://www.lotusmedical.org

Endnotes:

1. Wikipedia Foundation, Inc., The Hippocratic Oath, Online at (http://en.wikipedia.org/wiki/Hippocratic_Oath), (December 15, 2007).

2. Wikipedia, The Nightingale Pledge, Online at (http://en.wikipedia.org/wiki/NightingalePledge), (December 15, 2007).

3. Wikipedia, Physician, Online at (http://en.wikipedia.org/wiki/Physician), (December 15, 2007).

4. Wikipedia, Surgeon, Online at (http://en.wikipedia.org/wiki/Surgeon), (December 15, 2007).

5. Wikipedia, Physician, Online at (http://en.wikipedia.org/wiki/Physician), (December 15, 2007).

6. Mara Reinstein, "Tragic Loss," Us Weekly LLC, 1290, Avenue of the Americas, New York, Issue 668, December 3, 2007, pg 60.

7. "Cleveland Clinic Collaborates With Google to Enhance Patients' Healthcare Experience," The Cleveland Clinic, 02/20/2008 Online (http://cms.clevelandclinic.org/body.cfm?xyzpdqabc=0&id=227&action=detail&ref=815), (February 21, 2008).

8. Hilary Waldman, "Hartford Hospital on Probation," The Hartford Courant, Hartford, Hartford County, Connecticut, February 9, 2008, pg 1.

9. Lee Bowman, "Drug Names sound the same: A prescription for disaster," Scripps Howard News Service, as printed in the Waterbury Republican American, Waterbury, New Haven County, Connecticut, January 31, 2008. pg. 7A.

10. Alan Cohn, "Pharmacy Errors," WTNH Television Station, New Haven Co., New Haven, Connecticut, Team 8 Investigates, Aired July 19, 2002, 11:17 PM. EST.

11. "Kerry, Gingrich Tout E-Prescriptions To Cut Costs, Boost Quality," iHealth Beat, November 19, 2007, (http://www.ihealthbeat.org/), (November 19, 2007).

12. Michael Melia, "Tainted pills from Puerto Rico drug plants reach U.S," The Associated Press, Feb. 5, 2008, at 12:39 PM PST, online at: KOMO, Seattle Washington, TV/Health; (http://www.komotv.com/news/health/15366156.html), (2/5/2008).

13. Anna Boyd, "Chinese Heparin Factory Under Scrutiny, " 15:15, February 14, 2008, viewed online at eFluxMedia; (http://www.efluxmedia.com/news_Chinese_Heparin_Factory_Und er_Scrutiny_14013.html), (February 16, 2008).

14. United States Food and Drug Administration, " Information on Heparin Sodium Injection," FDA Web site. (www. FDA.gov.), dated March 18, 2008, (March 18, 2008).

15. United States Food and Drug Administration, "FDA's Drug Review and Approval Times," Last Updated: July 30, 2001, (http://www.fda.gov/cder/reports/reviewtimes/default.htm), (March 4, 2008).

16. Amy Goodwin interview with Dr. Sidney Wolfe, "Good Pills, Bad Pills: Dr. Sidney Wolfe Condemns FDA Advisors For Backing the Sale of Vioxx, Celebrex and Bextra Despite Known Dangers, Democracy Now, The War and Peace Report," Democracy Now Web site, February 22, 2005. Viewed online at: (http://www.democracynow.org/2005/2/22/good_pills_bad_pills_dr _sidney), (February 29, 2008).

17. Testimony script of Sidney M. Wolfe, M.D., "Congress Must Act Quickly to Address Growing Crisis At the Food and Drug Administration," PublicCitizen.org (www.citizen.org/pressroom/release.ccfm?ID=2617), (February 29, 2008).

18. Martha Raffaele, "Prescription-aid programs use "unsales" reps to steer away from high cost drugs," The Waterbury Republican American, Waterbury, New Haven County, Connecticut, March 3, 2008, pg 5a.

19. United States Environmental Protection Agency, "Pharmaceuticals and Personal Care Products," EPA Web site, (www.EPA.gov), updated March 10, 2008, (March 10, 2008).

20. Scott DeCarlo, Editor, Forbes.com, Inc., CEO Compensation, April 21, 2005, (www.forbes.com), (June 17, 2008).

21. Medical Billing Advocates of America, "Individual Services," online (www.billadvocates.com), (March 3, 2008).

22. Wikipedia, "Never Events," (www.en.wikipedia.org/wiki/Never_events), (March 1, 2008).

23. JoNel Aleccia, "Patients still stuck with bill for medical errors," MSNBC, February 29, 2008, (http://www.msnbc.msn.com/id/23341360/), (March 4, 2008).

24. The Associated Press, "59 People suing hospital, claiming abuse by doctor," The Waterbury Republican American, Waterbury, New Haven County, Connecticut, January 11, 2008, Pg. 3a.

25. Kohn L, ed, Corrigan J, ed, Donaldson M, ed., "Medical Mistakes Kill over 100,000 per year," To Err Is Human: Building a Safer Health System, Washington, DC: National Academy Press; 1999, on the Internet at: (http://www.mercola.com/1999/archive/medical_mistakes.htm) (December 17, 2007).

26. Ridgely Ochs and Michael Amon, "How Nurse led two hepatitis patients to one doctor," Newsday.com, Melville, N.Y., November 15, 2007, (www.newsday.com/ny-lihepa11115,0,5688574), (November 15, 2007).

27. Hillary Waldman, "Routine surgery, Fatal Error, Hospital Fined After Woman's Death," Courant.com, October 6, 2007, online at (www.topix.net/content/trb/2007/10/routine-surgery-fatal-error), (October 26, 2007).

28. "Endoscopy Center Closed by the City Today," By Sun Staff, The Las Vegas Sun, March 3, 2008, Online (http://www.natap.org/2008/newsUpdates/030308_04.htm), (February 29, 2008).

29. Winne Hu, "Manhattan Hospital is Fined After Cosmetic Surgery Deaths," The New York Times, May 16, 2004, online (http://query.nytimes.com/gst/fullpage.html?res=9506E7D7173FF93 5A25756C0A9629C8B63), (October 26, 2007).

30. "Medication Errors Injure 1.5 Million People and Cost Billions of Dollars Annually," The National Academies, Institute of Medicine Report, July 20, 2006, (http://www8.nationalacademies.org/onpinews/newsitem.aspx?Reco rdID=11623), (June 17, 2008).

31. Reuters, "Drug Name mix ups getting worse," Jan. 29, 2008, MSNBC, on the Internet at: (www. msnbc.msn.com/id/22901039/from/ET/), (February 6, 2008).

32. Pam Villarreal, "Malpractice system need radical reform," The Waterbury Republican-American, Waterbury, New Haven County, Connecticut, December 26, 2007. pg B3.

33. Christopher Lee, "Study Finds Gaps Between Doctors' Standards and Actions," Washington Post, December 4, 2007, pg AO8.

34. Chris Cuomo, News reporter, "Hospital Repeats Wrong Sided Brain Surgery," ABC Newscast, Aired November, 28, 2007, online at: (www.abcnews.go.com/Health), (November 30, 2007).

35. Reuters, "Half of Doctors mum about medical mistakes," December 3, 2007, online at: www.msnbc.msn.com , (www.msnbc.msn.com/id/22083982/print/1/displaymode/1098/), (12/17/2007).

36. Pam Villarreal, "Malpractice System needs radical Reform," The Waterbury Republican American, Waterbury, New Haven County, Connecticut, December 26, 2007. Online at: (http://www.rep-am.com/articles/2008/01/23/opinion/syndicated_columnists/306686.txt), (December 26, 2007).

37. Holtman, Matthew. "Disciplinary Careers of Drug-Impaired Physicians," Paper presented at the annual meeting of the American Sociological Association, Marriott Hotel, Loews Philadelphia Hotel, Philadelphia, PA, Aug. 12, 2005. Online at: (http://www.allacademic.com/meta/p18558_index.html), (February, 24, 2008).

38. American Association of Colleges of Nursing, Nursing Shortage Fact Sheet, Updated October 2007, online at: (http://www.aacn.nche.edu/Media/FactSheets/NursingShortage.htm) (January, 11, 2008).

39. American Association of College of Nursing, Nursing Shortage Fact Sheet, updated October 2007, online at: (www. aacn.nche.edu/Media/Factsheets/nursingshortage), (February 26, 2008).

40. American Association of Colleges of Nursing, Nursing Shortage Fact Sheet, Updated October 2007, online at: (http://www.aacn.nche.edu/Media/FactSheets/NursingShortage.htm) (January, 11, 2008).

41. IMS Health Incorporated, "IMS Reports U.S. Prescription Sales Jump 8.3 Percent in 2006, to $274.9 Billion," (http://www.imshealth.com/ims/portal/front/articleC/0,2777,6599_3 665_80415465,00.html), (March 1, 2008).

42. "Prescription Drugs and Senior Citizens," About.com: Tampa; The New York Times Company, on the Internet at: (http://tampa.about.com/od/governmentcityservices/i/prescripdrugs. htm), (February 18, 2008).

43. Walt Bogdanich, and Jake Hooker, "China Didn't Check Drug Supplier, Files Show," The New York Times, Published Feb. 16, 2008, Online at: (http://www.nytimes.com/2008/02/16/us/16baxter.html), (February 17, 2008).

44. "Verified Internet Pharmacy Practice Sites™ (VIPPS®)," The National Association of Boards of Pharmacy, On the Internet at: (www.nabp.net), (February 23, 2008).

45. "Patient Assistance Programs," NeedyMeds, Inc., Needymeds.com on the Internet at: (www.needymeds.com), (January 13, 2008).

46. "RXAssist, Patient Assistance Program Center," RXassist.com, on the Internet at (www.RXAssist.com), (February 1, 2008).

47.Medline Plus, "Managed Care," The U.S. National Library of Medicine and the National Institutes of Health, on the Internet at (http://www.nlm.nih.gov/medlineplus/managedcare.html), (August 20, 2008).

48. Stephanie Reitz, "Report: State needs more home services for elderly," The Waterbury Republican American, Waterbury, New Haven Co., Connecticut, published, January 12, 2008, pg 3a.

49. Geoffrey F. Joyce, Ph.D., Kanika Kapur, Ph.D., Krista A. Van Vorst, M.S., and Dr. Escarce, "Health Care Costs and Financing," on the Internet at (http://ahrq.hhs.gov/research/feb01/201RA15.htm); extracted from "Visits to primary care physicians and to specialists under gatekeeper and point-of-service arrangements," American Journal of Managed Care, November 6, 2000, pp. 1189-1196.

50. Wikipedia, "Managed Care," on the Internet at: (http://en.wikipedia.org/wiki/Managed_care), (December 17, 2007).

51. Wikipedia, "Hospital Medicine," online at: (http://en.wikipedia.org/wiki/Hospital_medicine), (February 1, 2008).

52. "New Specialty Serves Hospitalized Patients," Voices Weekender, Health Section, Prime Publishers Inc., Woodbury, Litchfield Co., Connecticut, February 10, 2008, pg 8.

53. Christopher Lee, "On call Specialists At Emergency Rooms Harder to Find, Keep," Washington Post, Friday, December 21, 2007, pg A1.

54. Sabrina Rubin Erdely, "Is your doctor playing judge?, " Self, June 2007, (www.self.com/livingwell.articles), (12/29/2007).

55. ibid.

56. U. S. Office of Personnel Management, Consumer Bill of Rights, online at: (http://www.opm.gov/insure/health/billrights.asp), (February 3, 2008).

57. HIPAA Rights, Fact Sheet, Protection and Advocacy for People with Disabilities, Inc., August 2005, on the Internet at: (http://www.protectionandadvocacy-sc.org), (2/1/2008).

58. Robert Gellman, "Health Privacy: The Way We Live Now," Version 1.1, Posted online at Privacyrights.org, Online at:(http://www.privacyrights.org/ar/gellman-med.htm), Posted: August 2002, viewed January 13, 2008.

59. "Hospital to Fire Worker in Spears Case," MSN Music News, March 14, 2008, online (http://music.msn.com/music/article.aspx?news+3054337&GT1=77 02), (March 16, 2008).

60. University of Connecticut Health Center, John Dempsey Hospital and UCONN Medical Group "Permission to Treat/Assignment of Benefits/Authorization to Release Medical Information/Acknowledgment of Receipt:Notice of Privacy Practices," Form HCH 901 Eff. 04/2003, revised 04/2006.

61. U.S. Department of State, "Tips for Traveling Abroad," Web site at: (http://travel.state.gov/travel/tips/tips_1232.html), (1/25/2008).

62. U.S. Department of State, "Health, What you need to Know in Advance of Travel," Web site at:(http://travel.state.gov/travel/tips/tips_1232.html#health), (1/25/2008).

63. Deborah Roberts and Nola Safro, "Cruise Lines are Responsible for Care Provided By Ship Doctors: Travel Myth or Fact?," ABC News, "20/20", Aired January 18, 2008, 10 P.M. EST.

64. Cruisebruise.com, "Janice Sullivan, Medical Malpractice of Ship's Doctor," Legend of the Seas - October 2005, Web site www.cruisebruise.com, online at: (www.cruisebruise.com/Janice_Sullivan.html), (12/18/2007).

65. Cruisebruise.com , "Edith Horn, Passenger Dies from Norovirus," MV Van Gogh, Travelscope Holidays - June 6, 2006, Web site www.cruisebruise.com, online at: (www.cruisebruise.com/Edith_Horn.html), 9 (12/18/2007).

66. Cruisebruise.com, "Janice Sullivan, Medical Malpractice of Ship's Doctor," Legend of the Seas - October 2005, Web site www.cruisebruise.com, online at: (www.cruisebruise.com/Janice_Sullivan.html), (12/18/2007).

67. Cruisebruise.com, "Helen Kerr, Medical Malpractice Results in Wrongful Death Carnival Legend," - September 6, 2006, Web site www.cruisebruise.com, online at: (www.cruisebruise.com/Helen_Kerr.html), (12/18/2007).

68. Cruisebruise.com, "Cruise Ship Medical Care Spotty, " Consumer Affairs.com , August 16, 2002, online at: (www.consumeraffairs.com/travel/cruise_safety.html), (12/18/2007).

69. David Krechevsky, "State cites Opticare for violations at surgical center," The Waterbury Sunday Republican, Waterbury, New Haven County, Connecticut, December 23, 2007. Page 1.

70.Trevor Thieme, "Ten Questions to Ask your Doctor," Best Life, on the Internet at: (http://health.msn.com), ((12/13/2007).

71. Associated Press, "Doctor given 3 years for liposuction death," Waterbury Republican American, Waterbury, New Haven County, Connecticut, March 19, 2008, pg. 5A.

72. "Unnecessary Operations," Prevention Health, viewed online at: (www.prevention.com/cda/article/unnecessary-operations/), (February 5, 2008).

73. Eric W. Nawar, M.H.S.; Richard W. Niska, M.D., F.A.C.E.P.; and Jianmin Xu, M.S., Division of Health Care Statistics, National Hospital Ambulatory Medical Care Survey: 2005 Emergency Department Summary, Center for Disease Control, June 29, 2007, (http://www.cdc.gov/nchs/data/ad/ad386.pdf), (March 3, 2008).

74. State of Connecticut, Connecticut Medical Examining Board, Minutes of Meeting, dated January 18, 2000, Petition number 980319-001-063. Online at (www.ct.gov/dph/lib/dph/phho/medical_board/minutes/connecticut_ medical_examining_board_2000_minutes.pdf), (December 17, 2007).

75. Catherine Winters, "I Was Exhausted All The Time," Ladies Home Journal, February 2008, Meredith Corporation, pg 140-144.

76. Courtney Hargrave, "Internal Affairs," Woman's Day Magazine, February 12, 2008, pg 56-57.

77. Julia Appleby,"Census: Health benefits scarcer," USA Today, Gannett Co., Inc., 8/28/2007. Viewed online at: (http://www.usatoday.com/money/industries/insurance/2007-08-28-uninsured_N.htm), (February 1, 2008).

78. National Academy of Sciences, "Uninsured Adults More Likely To Die Prematurely," News Release, May 21, 2002, online at: (http://www8.nationalacademies.org/onpinews/newsitem.aspx?RecordID=10367), (March 28, 2008).

79. FSA Feds, "What is the 'Use it or Lose it Rule'?," Web site; located at: (https://www.fsafeds.com/fsafeds/SummaryofBenefits.asp#WhatIsFSA) (January 2, 2008).

80. U. S. Treasury Department, "All About HSA's," published May 18, 2007.

81. The National Coalition on Health Care, "Facts on Health Insurance Coverage," online at: (http://www.nchc.org/facts/coverage.shtml), (June 4, 2008).

82. "Medical Bills Leading Cause of Bankruptcy, Harvard Study Finds," Consumer Affairs.com, February 3, 2005. Online at: (http://www.consumeraffairs.com/news04/2005/bankruptcy_study.html\), (December 22, 2007).

83. U. S Department of Labor, "Health Plans & Benefits, Continuation of Health Coverage - COBRA," On the Internet at: (http://www.dol.gov/dol/topic/health-plans/cobra.htm), (January 2, 2008).

84. Wikipedia, "HIPAA, Title I," Online at: (http://en.wikipedia.org/wiki/Health_Insurance_Portability_and_Accountability_Act) (November 26, 2007).

85. U. S. Department of Health Services, "Medicare, The Official U.S. Government Site for People with Medicare," Online at: (http://www.medicare.gov/MedicareEligibility/), (January 2, 2008).

86. Insure Me Web site, Insure Kids Now, available online at: (www.InsureKidsNow.net), (February 23, 2008).

87. The National Coalition on Health Care, "Facts on Health Insurance Coverage," online at: (http://www.nchc.org/facts/coverage.shtml), (June 4, 2008).

88. Wikipedia, "Managed Care," online at: (http://en.wikipedia.org/wiki/Managed_care), (December 15, 2007).

89. Wikipedia, "Managed Care," on the Internet at: (http://en.wikipedia.org/wiki/Managed_care), (December 17, 2007).

90. David M. Cutler, "Your Money or Your life: Strong Medicine for America's Health Care," Oxford University Press, 2004, 176 p.

91. Susan Haigh, "Healthy Lives might Garner Tax Breaks," Waterbury Republican American, Waterbury, New Haven County, Connecticut, February 28, 2008, pg A3.

92. Mary Jane Williams, RN, PhD., "Connecticut's Health Care Future: How can we improve access and affordability?" Connecticut Nursing News, Volume 80, Issue 4, December 2007, pg 10.

93. Richard Conniff, "How to Fix: Health Care," MSN Money, December 28, 2007, viewed online at: (http://articles.moneycentral.msn.com/Investing/HomeMortgageSavings/HowToFixHealthCare.aspx), (December 29, 2007).

94. State of Connecticut, Governor of Connecticut, "Governor Rell Announces $24.2 Million Federal Grant to Help Connecticut Residents Move from Nursing Homes," Released January 10, 2007, Office of Governor M. Jodi Rell, Governor of the State of Connecticut, viewed online at: http://www.ct.gov/governorrell/cwp/view.asp?A=2791&Q=330472, (January 15, 2008).

95. Carrie Macmillian, "Hearing Set on Medicaid Reform," Waterbury Republican American, Waterbury, New Haven County, Connecticut, March 2, 2008, Pg. 6 B.

96. U.S. Surgeon General, "My Family Health Portrait," U.S. Public Health Service Web page, online at : (https://familyhistory.hhs.gov/) (December 1, 2007).

97. Sandy Keefe, MSN, RN, "A Patient's Voice," Advance for Nurses, New England, December 17, 2007, pg 12.

98. Lacy BE, Rosemore J., Helicobacter pylori: ulcers and more: the beginning of an era. J Nutr. 2001;131:2789S–93S.

99. Linda A. Johnson, "Health Insurers limited Advanced Scans," viewed at Yahoo Finance at: (http://biz.yahoo.com/ap/080323/limiting_medical_scans.html?.v=4) (March 23, 2008).

100. Ibid.

101. "Increase Pay-up by Successfully Appealing Claim Denials," Appeal Solutions, Inc. (www.appealLettersOnline.com), (January 17, 2007).

102. Ben Popken, "As CIGNA Insurance waffles On Liver Transplant, Girl Dies," December 21, 2007, The Consumerist, (http://consumerist.com/search/As%20Cigna%20Insurance%20waffles%20on%20liver%20transplant,%20girl%20dies/), (December 22, 2007).

Index

347

348

349

350

355

About the Editor

Diane Ploch has worked in the communications field for 25 years and briefly in the medical field. She is an independent writer and marketing communications professional, running her own small business for 18 years. She has created communications projects in the venues of print, broadcast, video and the Internet. Her independent work is backed by experience as a public relations manager, newspaper reporter and story producer for a television magazine show. She has worked on projects covering various topics in health care, community service, manufacturing, corporate communications, politics and economic development. Diane holds a bachelor of science degree in Journalism from Southern Connecticut State University and an associate of applied science degree from Briarwood College, focusing on medical assisting. Diane lives in Southwestern Connecticut.